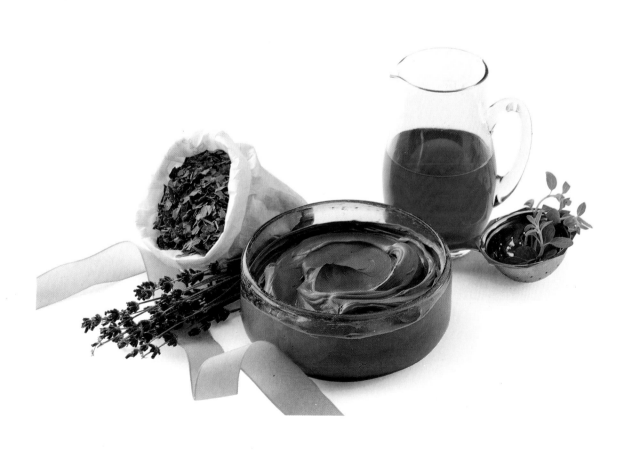

*For Raimondo Mattioli*

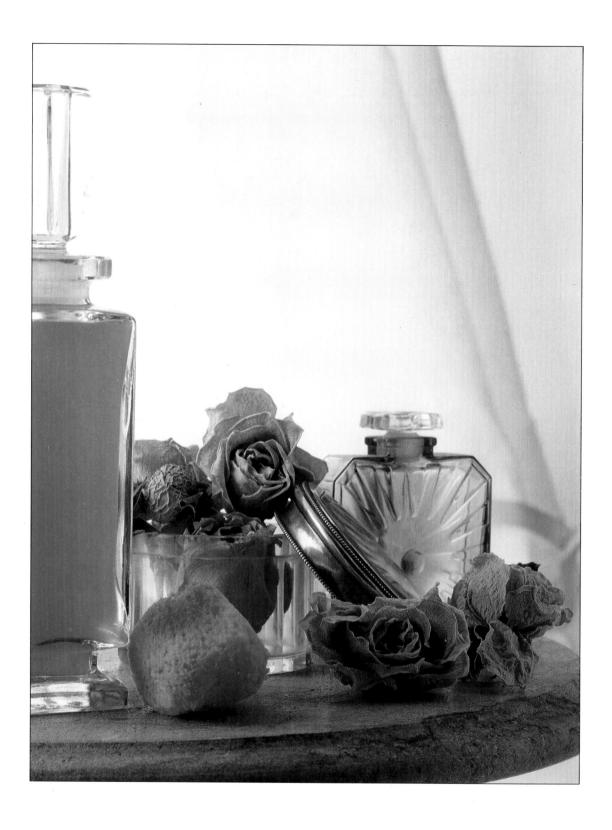

# NATURAL BEAUTY

Aldo Facetti

A Fireside Book
Published by Simon & Schuster Inc.
New York   London   Toronto   Sydney   Tokyo   Singapore

All the ingredients in the following recipes are measured by weight. Inexpensive, suitable scales are carried in most hardware stores, in health-food stores and herb shops, or can be bought from the mail-order suppliers listed at the back of this book.

Copyright © 1990 Arnoldo Mondadori Editore, S.p.A., Milan
English translation copyright © 1991 Arnoldo Mondadori Editore, S.p.A., Milan

English translation by Valerie Palmer

A Fireside Book
Published by Simon & Schuster Inc.
Simon & Schuster Building
Rockefeller Center
1230 Avenue of the Americas
New York, NY 10020

Fireside and colophon are registered trademarks of Simon & Schuster Inc.

Editor: Maria Luisa Viviani
Art Director: Giorgio Seppi
Cover Design: Simona Aguzzoni
Photographs by Chiara Madera, Milan

Typeset by Rowland Phototypesetting Ltd, Bury St Edmunds, Suffolk, England.
Printed and bound in Italy by Officine Grafiche Arnoldo Mondadori Editore, Verona.

10 9 8 7 6 5 4 3 2 1

**Library of Congress Cataloging in Publication Data**
Facetti, Aldo
  (Belle per natura. English)
  Natural beauty / Aldo Facetti; (English translation by Valerie Palmer)
    p.   cm.
  Translation of: Belle per natura.
  "A Fireside book."
  ISBN 0-671-74691-X
  1. Cosmetics.  2. Toilet preparations.  I. Title.
TP983.F313   1991
668'.55–dc20
                                                91–17495
                                                  CIP

# Contents

The author wishes to thank the following for their invaluable assistance and advise: Giovanni Agostini, Michele Artese, Giuseppe Borsati, Mario Carnero, Alessandro Del Carlo, Mario Giusti, Giovanni Lera, Angelo Lippi, Sirio Marconi, Riccardo Osini, Pierluigi Pannoli, Wanda Passadore, Mario Rosellini and Paolo Emilio Tomei.

# Introduction

*The purpose of this book is to show you how to make simple, homemade cosmetics, using natural ingredients, as an alternative to mass-produced products.*

*Not so long ago, every woman knew how to make creams and lotions from ordinary, everyday ingredients, using recipes which had been handed down for generations – the fruit of practical knowledge and experience.*

*To make a comparison with food, commercial cosmetics are to those you make yourself as fast food is to traditional home cooking. Just as you sometimes make good use of your free time by going back to the more laborious ways of preparing food, it is worth your time to make your own cosmetics. In the process, you will rediscover old recipes which are economical, effective and easy.*

*This book calls for a change of attitude regarding natural products. By using natural ingredients, you will be assured of products that are non-toxic, hypo-allergenic, fresh, and which can be "tailor-made" to suit your needs. Keep in mind, however, that* all *cosmetics – whether you prepare them yourself, or buy them in a store – should be used only as intended and kept out of the reach of children. Cosmetics* are for external use only, *and some natural ingredients – arnica, for example – are poisonous if drunk or ingested, even though they are perfectly safe and beneficial when applied externally and used according to the instructions in this book.*

*Many of the recipes in this book are based on old, traditional practices that can still be read today in the works of medieval alchemists and herbalists. I have reinterpreted them in light of twentieth-century knowledge and methods, and my hope is that by blowing off the dust of centuries I will have helped modern readers rediscover for themselves nature's secrets of personal hygiene and skin care.*

Aldo Facetti

# Basic ingredients

*The recipes in this book do not require a knowledge
of mysterious chemical substances. Most of the
ingredients are well known and readily available.
Some you may be able to find growing wild in the
countryside, others you can grow yourself in a
garden or window box. You can also buy herbs,
various oils, resins and waxes in specialized shops.
Other ingredients can be found in pharmacies or
health-food stores or from specialist suppliers.*

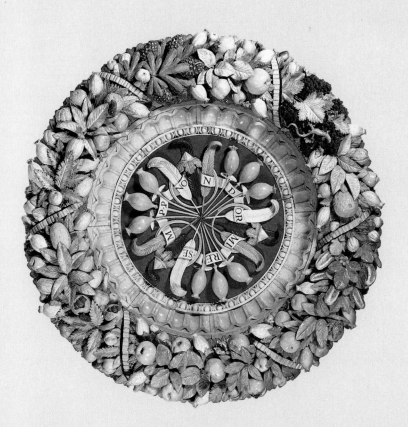

# Fresh ingredients

If you have plants that have been freshly gathered, their properties will be far more active than those you have dried or bought in a store.

If you grow annual plants, which complete their life cycle in autumn, you should dry them for use during the winter. A good book on herbs will tell you exactly when to harvest them and the best methods for drying and preserving the individual parts.

*Fir.* Over the centuries, various pagan rituals related to the winter solstice were assimilated into celebrations of the Nativity. The Christmas tree is a case in point: it was originally part of the ancient "cult of the tree," and had nothing to do with Christianity. Today, the Christmas tree is a source of yuletide cheer – but it also has cosmetic properties that most people ignore. If you are one of the millions of people who use a cut tree, do not throw it away after Christmas is over. The fragrant green buds and needles make a healthy, relaxing bath, and will help keep you healthy and invigorated throughout the winter.

*Orange.* As one of the last fruits of the year, the orange, with its sunny shape and bright colour, brings a touch of summer to the winter months. The peel has a subtle aroma and the sweet, succulent juices are tempered by just the right amount of acidity. The orange is also a source of vitamins and minerals that are highly beneficial. With the leaves, even of the bitter varieties which are usually only used as decoration, you can prepare a bath which will leave your skin soft and delicately perfumed. The essential oil found in the leaves, flowers and fruit is called neroli oil, after the Duchess of Neroli, who started a fashion for using it in the 1600s among the noble women of Rome.

*Marigold or* Calendula officinalis. This plant takes its names from the Latin word *calendae*, meaning the first day of the month, because it flowers in every month of the year, even in winter in areas where the

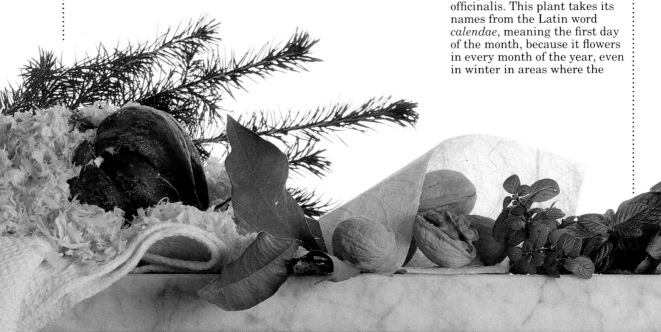

climate is mild. The flowers are like big, orange daisies and are used for a wide range of medicinal, cosmetic and culinary purposes. They can be gathered fresh, or dried in the shade.

*Eucalyptus.* This is the tallest tree in the world: in Australia, its native land, there are eucalyptus trees 500 feet (150 meters) tall. This beautiful, majestic tree grows very quickly and has dense, perennial foliage with a strong aroma. In the nineteenth century, it was believed that eucalyptus could disinfect areas infested with malaria.

*Juniper.* This tree has pointed green needles and green and black berries. The berries are used to flavour traditional game dishes, succulent roasts, rich meat stews, smoked meats and sauerkraut. Their distinctive taste has long been appreciated and they have been used in flavoured liqueurs and spirits, the most familiar of which is gin (which takes its name from the first three letters of *ginepro*, the Italian word for juniper).

*Mint.* This is the most instantly recognizable of all the herbs and medicinal plants used since ancient times. Its very name bears witness to its history.

According to Greek mythology, Minthe was a beautiful nymph loved by Pluto, the god of the underworld. His wife Persephone, mad with jealousy, turned Minthe into a little plant. Its mythical derivation and intense perfume convinced some ancient cultures that this plant was a powerful aphrodisiac, and medieval sorcerers and alchemists placed it under the sign of Venus.

*Walnut.* This plant has long been associated with the gods – Linnaeus, the father of modern botany, called it "Jove's acorn" – and with the occult. It figured in strange rituals during which wizards and witches supposedly assembled at full moon beneath a walnut tree. Because of its resemblance to the human brain, the fruit of the tree has also given rise to all kinds of stories and beliefs, both in

folklore and medieval medicine.

*Laurel or Bay.* Like an impoverished nobleman whose name perpetuates the memory of former glories, the Latin name for this handsome tree, *Laurus nobilis*, bears witness to its illustrious past. In the Greek and Roman world, it was dedicated to Apollo, the god of sunlight, music, poetry and prophecy, and was worn as an emblem of literary or military achievement.

*Basil.* "Fit for the house of a king" is the meaning of the name for this plant, derived from the ancient Greek. Basil comes from India, and undoubtedly owes its name to its powerful aroma. It is used in a number of famous food recipes, including Italian *pesto* sauce and the French *soupe au pistou*, a vegetable soup with garlic and herbs.

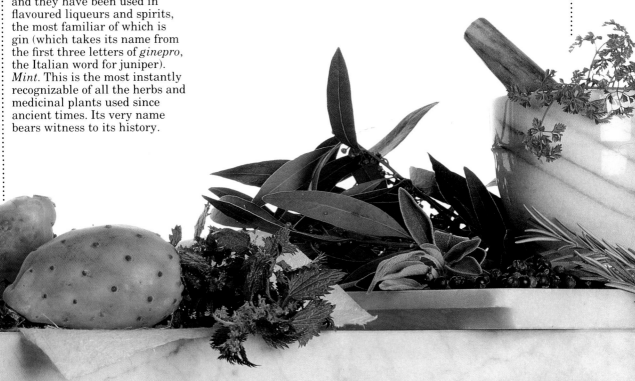

# Dried herbs

Herbs should be picked at the point when they contain the highest concentration of active principles. They should be dried immediately, or they will soon deteriorate. Each plant has its own optimum period for picking. This will be indicated in any good herbal guide. Whether in the shade, sun or oven, the best drying method for the different parts (flowers, leaves, roots, bark) will also be described in a good book. Humidity, light and time are the three reasons plants lose their active principles.
*Aniseed.* The seeds of this richly aromatic herb are used in

confectionery, breadmaking and home cooking. The essential oil which produces their tempting aroma is a valuable aid to health and beauty too.
*Chamomile.* This is one of the most time-honoured medicinal herbs, symbolic of a tradition based on the collective wisdom of generations for preparing simple, home-made remedies – a tradition which is well worth reviving. It has long been used internally as a mild sedative and in connection with stomach disorders. It has also been used externally for rashes, skin inflammations and skin protection against the elements.
*St. John's wort.* The botanical name for this plant, *Hypericum perforatum*, is indicative of the peculiarity of its leaves, sepals and petals. If you hold them up

against the light, they appear to be covered in translucent spots, like perforations. St. John's wort was named after the order of knights who, during the Crusades, hung it around their horses on St. John's Eve to ward off evil spirits. People also used to hang it outside their houses, or wear it as a charm to protect them from the evil eye. Picked before dawn and eaten, it was thought to cure rabies and mental illnesses inflicted by the devil. Recent studies have shown that St. John's wort is an excellent remedy for skin complaints. The traditional red oil recipe is an effective treatment for minor cuts and abrasions, and for mild cases of

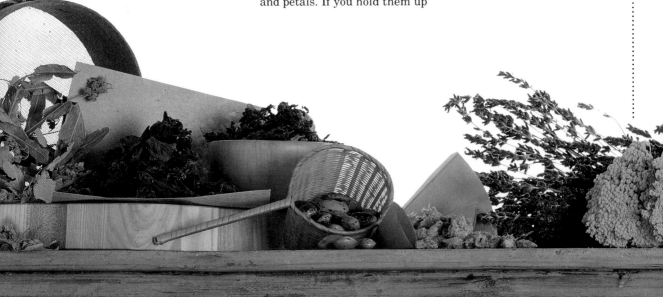

sunburn. It is even a good anti-wrinkle treatment.

*Lavender.* This plant has been used since ancient times and occupies a special place in popular tradition. The name comes from the Latin word *lavare*, "to wash," as lavender was added to bath water and laundry for its fresh, clean smell. This sun-loving Mediterranean plant thrives in hot, dry areas. The unmistakeable aroma is a distinctive feature of the Mediterranean *maquis* with its characteristic blend of perfumes. Lavender is an adaptable plant, however, and has adjusted to the more humid, misty conditions of the northern climates to which it has been introduced, without losing its perfume. In fact, the best lavender nowadays is said to come from plants grown in England. Lavender is full of essential oil which is very good for the skin, and also acts as an insect repellent. The flowers contain the most oil.

*Flax.* Ancient Chinese, Peruvian, Egyptian and Mesopotamian civilizations all made use of this valuable plant. Linen made with it has been used for thousands of years, and is still one of the best fabrics available. Our ancestors would fill huge chests and closets with handspun linen, which was repeatedly washed and left out in the sun to bleach out the natural colour. Young girls would spend countless hours turning the material into sheets, towels, tablecloths and curtains, hemming and embroidering with great care. Linen was used for special occasions. The tablecloth for the feast, towels for the distinguished guest or the visiting doctor, the sheet for the bridal bed – all were proudly displayed for their dazzling whiteness. Flax is not just valued for its fiber. Its seeds (linseed) are made into flour and oil, both of which are used in the preparation of cosmetics.

*Marsh mallow.* In the light of modern knowledge, this humble plant can no longer be regarded as a panacea for all ills, as it once was. But it is a useful treatment for some minor ailments, because of its anti-inflammatory properties. Marsh mallow grows wild in many parts of North America and Europe, and the only cost involved is that of picking it. If you have a garden or vegetable plot, grow some marsh mallow there, so that it is always at hand. Pick the leaves off one by one, without the stalks; they will soon grow again. Marsh mallow is very good for many different skin irritations. It is a powerful emollient, which softens and nourishes the skin and mucous membranes.

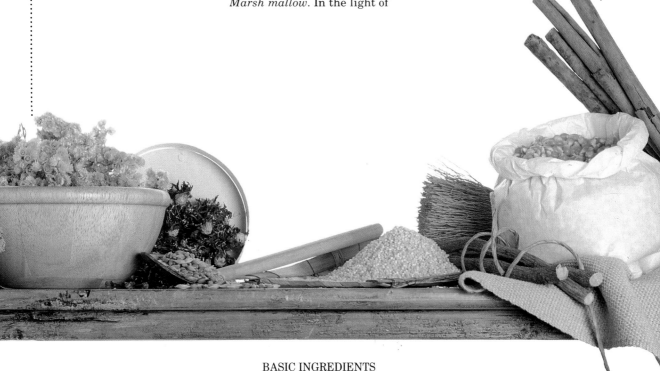

# Fruit and vegetables

At the dawn of time, succulent fruit and vegetables and soft, tender leaves must have been the primary sources of cleansing and healing materials, along with water and saliva. These would have been the first dressings applied to skin injuries inflicted by thorns, rough tree bark and rocks, and even the teeth and claws of wild animals. In time, over the course of thousands of years, different civilizations discovered additional cosmetic uses for the pulp and juices of edible fruits and vegetables.

The first rule in using fruits and vegetables is that they must not be damaged or show any signs of decomposition. If they are not fit to eat, they are not fit to make cosmetics from. But remember that it is the inside that counts, not the exterior: a wild apple with a few wormholes may spoil your appetite, but not its use as a cosmetic ingredient.

Nowadays there are far too many vitamins, minerals and trace elements sold in pill-form. Unless they have been prescribed by a doctor, it is much better to assimilate vitamins and minerals directly from the foods which contain them: seasonal fruit and vegetables and other "live" foods like yogurt, honey, molasses, yeast and wheatgerm. Remember that beauty depends on health and that you really *are* what you eat! Nearly all fruits contain vitamin A, B1, B2 and C, and many have B3 and B6 as well. The other vitamins are not found in such reliable quantities, but if you eat a variety of seasonal foods throughout the year, you will cover the full range of vitamins, minerals and trace elements needed for good health and beauty.

*Grapes.* The end of summer and the glorious colours of autumn have been associated since time immemorial with the pagan ritual of the grape harvest. It is a ceremonial occasion that seems almost to exorcise all thoughts of the dark, cold winter ahead, and that provides a warm drink of sunshine in the cold, gloomy months to come.

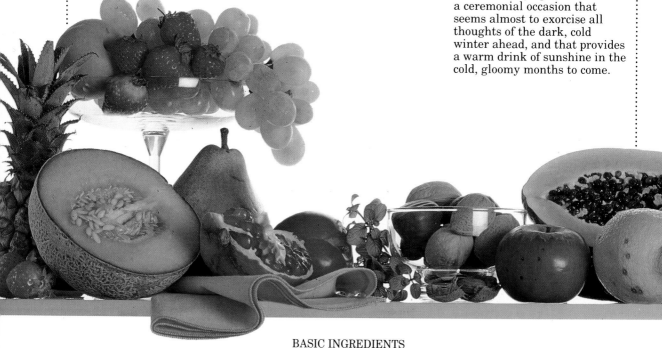

The people of wine-growing countries have a primeval relationship with the fruit of the vine. It has long been regarded as a living, vital substance, a type of blood in vegetable form – a conception that in some sense is true because of the enzymes it contains. The medical and cosmetic value of the vine comes from hundreds of years of observing the effects of its leaves, tendrils, bark, sap, grape, juice, wines and spirits.

*Carrot.* For beautiful skin, thick, shiny hair, sparkling eyes, slim hips, muscle tone and vitality, you should eat carrots daily. You can eat them raw, add them to salads, or make them into a refreshing drink using a juice extractor. Carrot juice is an excellent tonic, which is easily absorbed and very low in calories. Try drinking it at breakfast, mixed with orange, lemon or grapefruit juice and garnished with a slice of kiwi fruit, or as an aperitif, mixed with tomato juice and garnished with a fresh basil leaf. Carrot juice forms the basis of some good vitamin and tonic treatments for the skin.

*Cabbage.* Raw cabbage juice or boiled and chopped cabbage leaves can be used for face masks which soften and refine the skin and are particularly good for oily, acne-prone skin. You can also drink the juice and eat the raw chopped leaves lightly boiled or in salads.

*Watermelon, musk melon, cucumber and marrow or squash.* These are all members of the family of Cucurbitaceae, and share the same thirst-quenching properties. The juices are so refreshing that you can literally eat, drink and wash your face with them! Once again, popular understanding is borne out by modern research, which has shown that the flesh and juices – which are mildly astringent (particularly cucumber) or emollient (melon and squash) – have a high vitamin and mineral salt content. They are one of the most refreshing items in summer and are very good for the skin. For those who lead an outdoor life with skin exposed to sun and wind, this family will help treat redness, inflammation, wrinkles and other signs of premature ageing.

*Cherry.* Bright red cherries suspended from stalks like wishbones, or hooked over ears like baubles are among the happy memories of childhood – though their firm, succulent flesh and mouthwatering taste are probably most keenly remembered. They are healthy to eat, and the flesh can be crushed and used as a face mask.

*Apple.* Aside from its unfortunate role in the garden of Eden, there is really nothing bad that one can say about this fruit. Many different cultures have a proverb to the effect that "an apple a day keeps the doctor away"; in addition, this fruit has cosmetic properties that have been exploited for centuries. For example, the pomade – a hair preparation popular in the seventeenth and eighteenth centuries – was named after the apple (*pomata* in Italian). It will help keep the skin of the whole body fresh and healthy, and is especially good at clearing facial complexion.

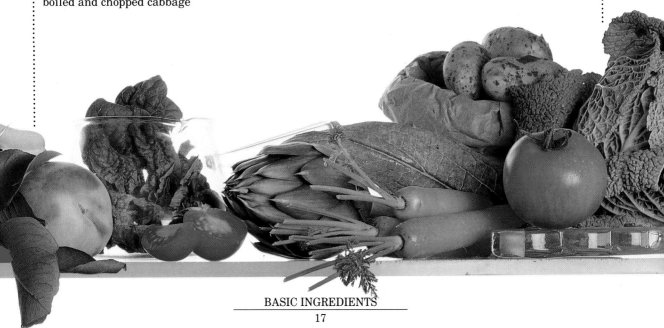

# Other ingredients

This is just a small selection from the enormous range of natural substances our ancestors used on their skin, believing the foods which endowed them with health and strength must contain hidden beauty secrets. Why not experiment with other foods to see what new recipes for beautiful skin and hair you can devise?

*Vinegar.* Vinegar comes from the acetous fermentation of alcoholic beverages (wine, cider, beer, etc.) by microorganisms of the genus *Acetobacter*. Different types of vinegar (wine, cider, malt, etc.) have been used in cosmetics since ancient times, either alone or with aromatic plants, flowers, fruit, essential oils, alcoholic tinctures or resins (medicinal or aromatic vinegars). They have been used neat or diluted with water as skin toners and mouthwashes; as rinses to make the hair soft and shiny after washing; as antiseptics, deodorants and for general refreshment.

*Clay.* Clay consists of minute particles of siliceous rocks (granites and feldspars) which were carried along by rivers and streams in previous geological eras and deposited in huge masses, now excavated. During their journey through the earth, these minerals were enriched with trace elements which dyed them different colours. The clays may be green, red or white, and their properties will vary according to the elements they contain. Clay has been used for health and beauty treatments since time immemorial – in mud baths, or as face packs. One type of North

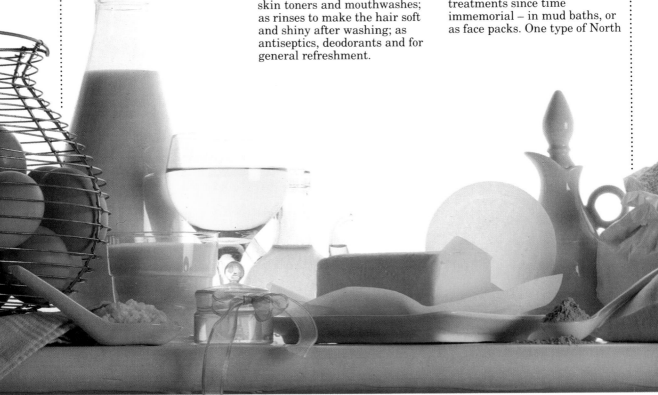

African clay, rhassoul mud, is used to clean the hair.

*Molasses*. Molasses is a by-product of the refining of sugar cane. This thick, dark, honey-like substance is packed with vitamins and minerals and is used for dietary and cosmetic purposes.

*Malt*. Malt is produced by the partial germination of cereal grains. During this process, the starch in the seeds turns to sugars rich in enzymes, salts and vitamins. It comes in the form of a thick syrup, similar to honey, and is used for breadmaking and in cosmetics.

*Maple*. Maple syrup is obtained from the concentrated sap of the sugar maple, or *Acer saccarum*, a common North American tree. Used as a sweetener, it is rich in sugars, minerals salts and vitamins. Its cosmetic uses are similar to those of honey, malt and molasses.

*Aqua vitae*. This is an old-fashioned name for spirits distilled from the pressed juice (fermented must) of fruit, cereals, syrups and even wine, cider and other moderately alcoholic beverages. They have different names, depending on their countries of origin and methods of production: brandy, grappa, cognac, whisky, vodka, etc. Like vinegar, they are also used in cosmetics to make extracts, perfumes and lotions.

*Cocoa butter*. Cocoa butter is obtained from the seeds of the cocoa plant, which are 40–50% composed of this fatty substance. It has a long history of use in confectionery, pharmaceutical, and cosmetic industries. It is a particularly effective emollient (softening and soothing agent) which protects the skin and mucous membranes.

*Beeswax*. Bees process honey and turn it into wax at the rate of one pound of wax for every ten pounds of honey. The bees use it in hives to make honeycombs with hexagonal cells. A bee larva is put in each compartment, together with pollen and honey, and the cells are then closed with a thin layer of wax. The wax from these structures is of particular value in cosmetics.

*Honey*. Apart from being highly nutritious, honey is an effective treatment for cuts and wounds. It soothes skin irritations and is mild enough to be used on children's skin. Because it is so good for the skin, it is included in numerous recipes for creams, balms, lotions and face masks.

*Propolis or bee glue*. This is a brown, resinous substance collected by bees from the buds of trees. The bees use it to paint the insides of the hives, and to mummify the bodies of any intruders. Its disinfectant properties make it a good natural antibiotic for local use. It is effective against bacterial or fungal infections of the skin, as an antiseptic applied to minor wounds, and in the treatment of outer mouth inflammations. It also acts as an analgesic and anti-irritant.

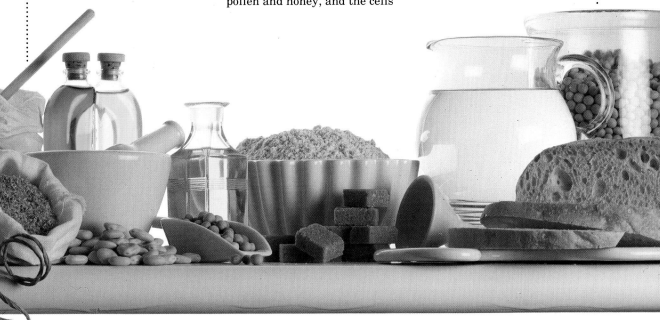

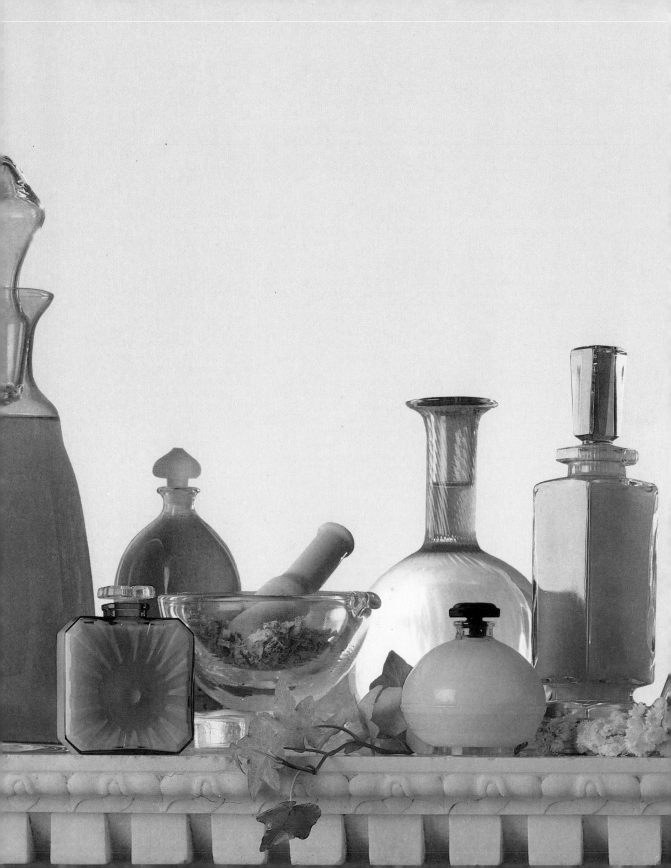

# Basic preparations

*Pharmacists of the past have been described as brilliant chefs, because of their resourcefulness in preparing elixirs, electuaries, pomades, lotions and potions. We can all seek to emulate them nowadays, as the modern kitchen is equipped with a range of gadgetry beyond the wildest dreams of the alchemists. Just follow the recipes and watch the magic unfold.*

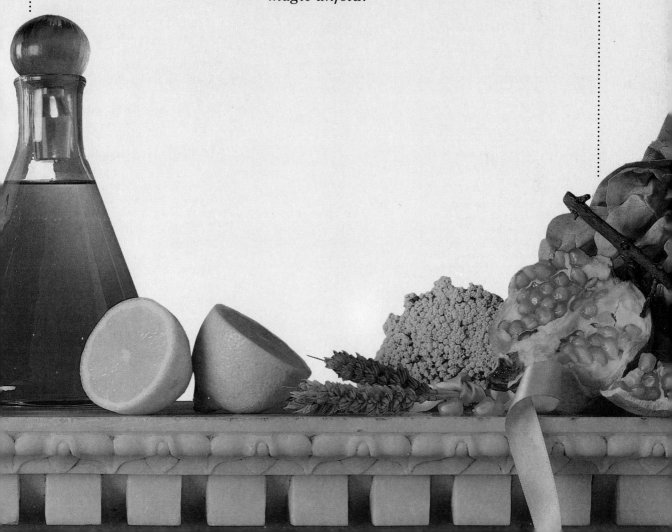

## Preparation rules

All the cosmetics in this book are completely free of preservatives, bacterial agents, antifungal agents and antioxidants. This means that, like food, they will only keep for a limited period. You can increase their lifespan by using the same techniques as you would to prevent food from spoiling: use spotlessly clean containers and implements and keep the containers covered. The cosmetics will keep a few days longer if you refrigerate them, and 2–3 months if you freeze them.

It is always best to use new bottles for storage. If they are used ones, wash them thoroughly and then sterilize them by boiling in water for 20 minutes, particularly if they have contained liquids other than water or alcohol. Pots and jars for creams should be treated in the same way. Remember also when using the cream, never dip your fingers into a jar: use the tip of a knife or teaspoon, which will contaminate the mixture less.

Many recipes include the use of a blender in the instructions as this is the best way to make the smoothest and most amalgamated products. If you do not have a blender, food processor, electric whisk, etc., equally good results can be obtained by beating meticulously, crushing with a pestle and mortar or with the back of a rolling pin, according to the recipes' ingredients and textures required.

As well as some basic kitchen equipment, such as bowls, jugs, tablespoons and teaspoons, you will need a good pair of scales to measure the ingredients accurately.

# LEAF BUDS MACERATED IN GLYCERINE

*This process serves to extract valuable, active substances from the buds of trees and shrubs. These are preserved in glycerine, then used in cosmetics.*

*The buds contain the leaves, branches, flowers and fruit which develop from them, in embryonic form. Like seeds, they therefore contain the highest concentration of active nutrients in the entire plant.*

*The recipe here is for cosmetic use – not for medical use. The technique was pioneered by the Belgian physician Pol Henry in the 1950s. He based it on his theory that the growth tissues of plants contained special substances with strong therapeutic properties.*

## Collecting the buds.

*The buds should be collected in late winter or early spring, before they open. At this point they contain the highest concentrations of active nutrients.*

*Make sure that the plants are not near any obvious source of pollution. Ideally they should be as far away as possible from towns, heavy industry or busy roads. Even in the countryside, constant traffic and intensive farming methods involving the use of pesticides can affect nearby plants, so you will need to watch out for this.*

*Prune some small branches, take them home, and cut off the buds, using a small, stainless steel knife.*

*Discard any imperfect buds and wash the others under cold tap water.*

*The following recipe uses lime/ linden buds as an example.*

## Method of preparation

*Maceration generally involves steeping a plant or part of a plant in a solvent, at room temperature in an airtight container.*

*The solvent can be water, oil, alcohol, wine, vinegar, glycerine, etc., according to the purpose for which it is intended.*

# Leaf buds macerated in glycerine

## INGREDIENTS

⅓ oz/10 g fresh lime/linden buds

7 oz/200 g anhydrous glycerine

3½ oz/100 g alcohol at least 60°
proof (e.g. vodka, brandy). Do *not*
use treated alcohol such as
surgical or industrial spirit or
ethyl alcohol.

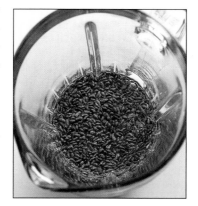 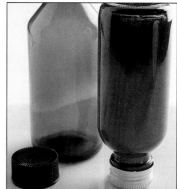

*Put the buds and glycerine in a
blender and blend for a minute at
low speed and a minute at high
speed.*

•

*Pour the mixture into a dark glass
bottle, filling it to the brim. Seal and
leave to macerate for two weeks at
room temperature, shaking the bottle
daily.*

•

*Transfer the mixture to a larger
bottle and add the spirits. Leave for
one more week, still shaking daily.*

•

*Strain the liquid through a fine,
stainless steel or plastic sieve.*

•

*Pour into clean, dark glass bottles,
filling them to the brim, and store in
a cool dark place, not the
refrigerator. The mixture should
keep for at least three years, and can
be added to creams, cleansing milks
and some face masks.*

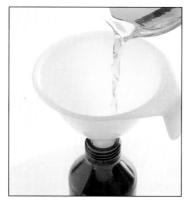 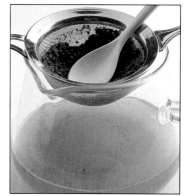

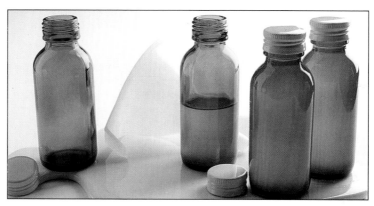

## MOTHER TINCTURE

*The active elements of medicinal plants undergo changes over time, and consequently their quality deteriorates with age. This is a problem for which various solutions have been tried through the centuries. One successful technique involves making extracts using the ethyl alcohol in wine or brandy. The alcohol is an effective solvent, and also acts as a preservative. Techniques for making medicines from herbs were refined in the monasteries of Europe in the Middle Ages. The herbs were steeped in quality wines. Later, liquids with a higher percentage of alcohol, known as* aqua vitae *(literally, the water of life, or the elixir of life), were used for this process. These medicinal liquors were administered to travel-weary pilgrims, or to soldiers recovering from battle during the Crusades.*

*At the beginning of the nineteenth century, the German physician Samuel Hahnemann, who founded homeopathy, invented the term "mother tincture" to refer to alcoholic tinctures of fresh herbs, from which many homeopathic medicines are derived.*

*Even though the expression "mother tincture" is used in recipes for cosmetic use, the procedures for making them are much simpler than those used for homeopathic ones.*

*If you prefer not to make your own tinctures, homeopathic versions are available from pharmacies and herbalists, but remember to halve the amounts stated in the recipes.*

# Mother tincture of fresh herbs

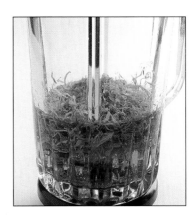

## INGREDIENTS

1½ oz/40 g freshly picked marigold flowers

3½ oz/100 g alcohol at least 60° proof (e.g. vodka, brandy). Do *not* use treated alcohol such as surgical or industrial spirit or ethyl alcohol.

Ratio of plant to solvent 2:5.

*For an alternative version using dried herbs at a plant-to-solvent ratio of 1:10, the ingredients are:*

⅓ oz/10 g dried chamomile flowers

3½ oz/100 g alcohol

*Chop the fresh or dried flowers finely, using a two-handled blade and plastic chopping board or a pestle and mortar. Reduce to a pulp if fresh or a powder if dry. Mix with the alcohol. Alternatively, pour all the ingredients into a blender and run it for a minute at low speed and a minute at high speed.*
•

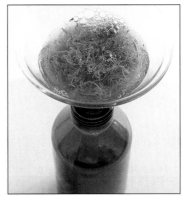

*Fill an airtight, dark glass bottle with the mixture to the brim to prevent oxidization.*
•

*Leave in a dark place for three weeks, shaking daily. Strain, first through a sieve, squeezing out the liquid, then through a paper filter. Pour into small, dark glass bottles, filling to the brim. Make sure they are clean and airtight. They should be stored in a cool, dark, dry place, not the refrigerator. The tincture will keep for three years.*

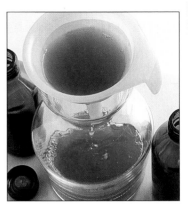

## PLANTS MACERATED IN OIL

*This technique is used to extract the volatile essential oils from aromatic herbs. The oils are released by the plants when they are immersed in an oily solvent at room temperature.*

*The most suitable solvent is virgin olive oil, which keeps better than other types. The next best is sweet almond oil. Other oils extracted from crushed seeds without using solvents are also acceptable (e.g. peanut, sunflower, corn, soya, grapeseed).*

*The ratio of plant to oil is usually 1:5, but the amount of oil can be increased, especially if you macerate more than one herb in the same oil.*

*Maceration takes from one to three weeks. Extraction is quickened if the airtight container is exposed to gentle heat (86°–95°F/30°–35°C). The more finely the plant is chopped, the more rapidly and completely it will release its active principles.*

*Stronger aromatic oils can be obtained by repeating the process several times.*

*After a plant has been steeped in oil long enough for it to have released its active principles, it will be "exhausted." It should then be replaced by a fresh dose. You can do this three or four times, until the oil is saturated with aroma.*

*The following two recipes are for St. John's wort oils but they are also the basic recipes for other plant oil.*

# Dr. Leclerc's oil of St. John's wort

### INGREDIENTS

3½ oz/100 g flower heads of St. John's wort (*Hypericum perforatum*)

3½ oz/100 g dry white wine

7 oz/200 g virgin olive oil

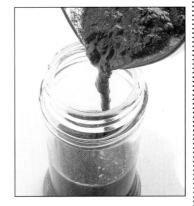

*Blend the ingredients in a blender for a minute at low speed and a minute at high speed.*

•

*Pour the contents into a wide-mouthed glass jar; steep for three days at room temperature, shaking the jar twice daily.*

•

*Heat the mixture in a double boiler until all the wine has evaporated.*

•

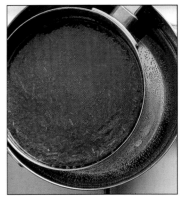

*When tepid, pour through a strainer and then filter paper. Squeeze out the mixture and fill dark glass bottles with the liquid to the brim. The bottles should have airtight lids. This crimson-coloured oil is similar to the one in the following recipe, obtained by steeping the herbs in the sun.*

*If you do not have the time to prepare macerated oils or cannot obtain the fresh or dried plants, you can buy them at herbalists or health-food stores.*

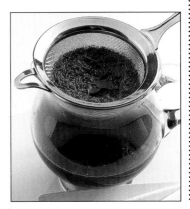

# St. John's wort oil

### INGREDIENTS

3½ oz/100 g flower heads of
St. John's wort

1 lb 2 oz/500 g virgin olive oil

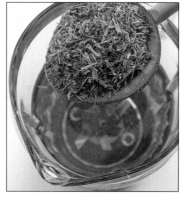
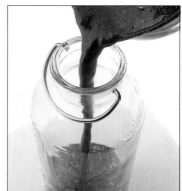

*Freshly-picked St. John's wort flower heads and leaves are small enough to absorb oil readily. Cut them off with stainless-steel scissors. Mix well with the olive oil to extract the essential oil. You can do it in a blender for a minute at low speed and a minute at high speed.*

•

*Transfer the ingredients to a wide-mouthed jar, seal and leave in the sun for three weeks, shaking daily. The resulting oil will be red.*

•

*To improve the product, remove the used flower heads from the oil, squeeze them out or let them drip, and replace with other, freshly-picked flower heads. Repeat the instructions above.*

•

*Filter the oil, first through a fine sieve and then through filter paper, cheesecloth, or double muslin bag. Squeeze out the mixture. Discard*

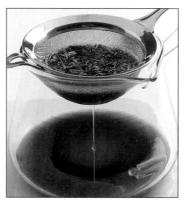
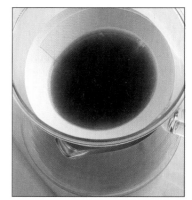

*watery liquid, sap and plant juices at the bottom. You only need the oil.*

•

*Pour into clean, screw-top dark glass bottles. The oil will keep better if you use several small bottles rather than one big one.*

•

*The same process can be used for yarrow, marigold and chamomile flowers, and for bay, marjoram, rosemary and thyme leaves. Two macerations are quite enough for all of these.*

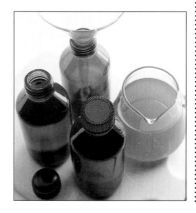

# Infusion

This is the same process used for making a cup of tea. It serves to extract aromatic or water-soluble active principles from leaves, flowers and seeds.

A generous teaspoon of finely-chopped herbs is added to a cup of water, after this has been brought to a boil in a stainless steel saucepan. Use the purest water available, such as bottled mineral water (still water, not sparkling).

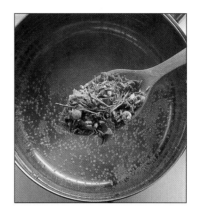

- Remove from the heat immediately and cover. Let stand for at least 10 minutes, then strain and sweeten with honey if required.

- When making infusions, the herbs must not be boiled. Important properties, such as the aromatic oils, would disperse with the steam, and certain vitamins and active principles are unstable when exposed to heat.

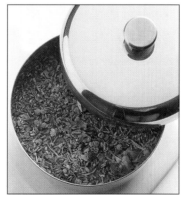

- Infusions can be kept for 24 hours in a sealed container in the refrigerator, but are best freshly made. They will keep frozen for a few weeks in airtight plastic containers.

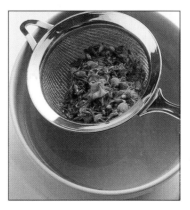

# Filtration

This process separates a liquid from the particles suspended in it. Plastic or stainless steel sieves are recommended for basic filtration.

- To obtain a reasonably clear liquid, make a cotton, cheesecloth or muslin filter shaped like a conical bag, which can be squeezed out at the end. You can fasten it to the inside of a funnel with paperclips.

- For small amounts of liquid which are not too dense or viscous, you can line a sieve or strainer with a layer of cotton wool/cotton, although paper filters give the clearest results.

- Paper filters are available at pharmacies, hardware and health-food stores. Choose the proper density, depending on how clear a liquid is needed, and whether they are to be used for water, alcohol or oil. Some have folds which make them easier to fit into funnels and support the weight of the ingredients. The folds also help retain solid particles.

- To avoid splitting the paper, always pour the liquid a little at a time, against one side. To prevent clogging, filter the mixture through a sieve, muslin or cheesecloth first.

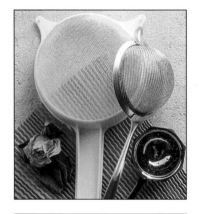
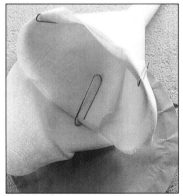
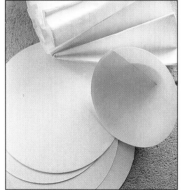
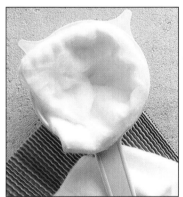
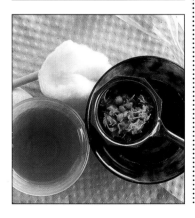

# Decoction

# Bain-marie

*This is a method to extract water-soluble active principles from roots, bark wood, seeds, etc. It consists of boiling the ingredients in water, in a stainless steel saucepan over a very low heat. They should be thoroughly crushed. The water should be as pure as possible, ideally bottled, non-sparkling mineral water.*

•

*The minimum quantity you can use is the same as for infusions: a teaspoon. The amount of water needed is proportional to the preparation time: the longer you boil it, the more water you will need.*

•

*For the best results, soak the ingredients for several hours beforehand, as you would to shorten the cooking time for dried peas, beans, lentils, etc.*

•

*Decoctions, like infusions, are best freshly prepared. They will keep for up to three days if refrigerated and for a few weeks in the freezer if placed in airtight plastic containers as soon as you have made them.*

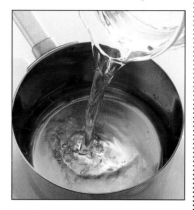

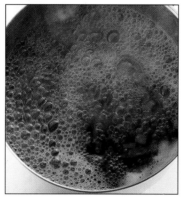

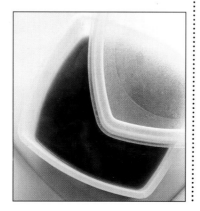

*This is a technique for heating or cooking something at no more than 212°F (100°C) using a double boiler.*

•

*Two containers are needed in this process. Use either a normal double boiler or a bowl immersed in a larger saucepan half-filled with water. The water is brought to a boil in the outer container; the inner one holds the ingredients to be heated.*

•

*Whatever heat setting you choose, the water will never exceed its own boiling point of 212°F (100°C), which it will transfer to the inner container.*

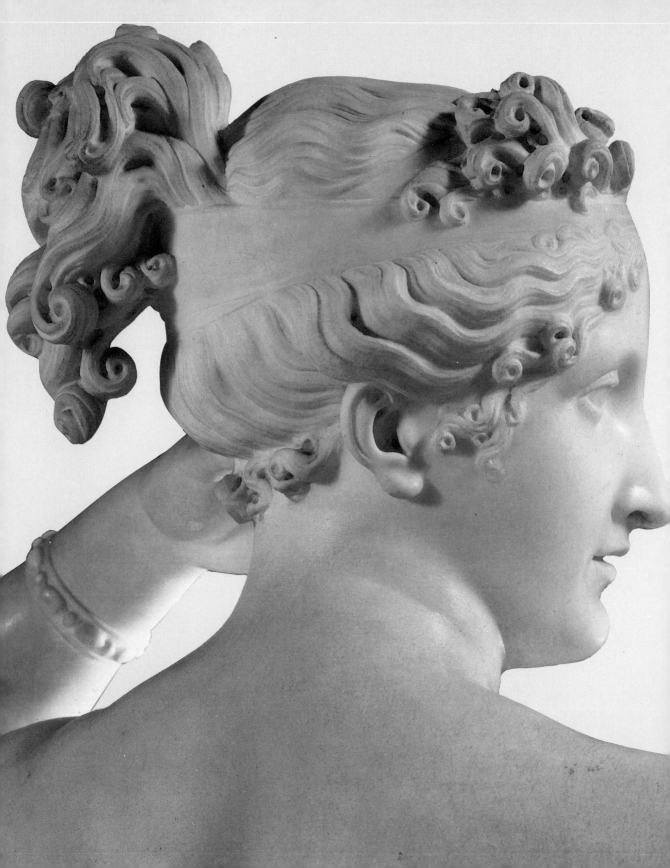

# The hair

*Hair has always been regarded as a reflection of beauty, health and strength – a crowning glory. Those who have it tend to flaunt it; those who do not wish they could!*
*Hair, nails and skin are the screen on to which our mental and physical well-being is projected. The cosmetics recommended here will help restore and maintain the balance and integrity of your hair.*

*M*ost minor hair problems nowadays are due to overwashing and excessive shampoo use. Overwashing often causes the scalp to react by producing more oil, a condition known as reactive seborrhea. It can be avoided by using natural shampoos, which are less aggressive. Reduce the amount of commercial shampoo you use and dilute it, or before each shampoo rub in an aromatic oil or a mixture of oils.

*It makes sense to avoid drastic hair treatments which use either chemicals or heat: these can damage the structure of the hair. Conditioners, balsams, lacquers, animal or vegetable gums can also upset the natural balance. Finally, do not forget that hair and fingernails are often the first parts of the body to tell you that something is wrong; you may not be ill, but pay attention to the alarm bell.*

*Avoid the mistake many make of thinking that hair is like grass and the more you "prune" it and the more "fertilizer" you put on it, the thicker and faster it will grow. The only ones likely to benefit from such treatment are the hair salons and the companies selling the products. The fact is that a well-balanced diet, including fresh seasonal foods, is the best insurance policy that there is for guaranteeing strong hair and nails.*

# Neutral henna scalp treatment

*This treatment strengthens hair, adds body, and controls dandruff and excess oiliness.*

### INGREDIENTS

2 oz/50 g neutral henna

12½ oz/350 g still mineral water

4 tsp/20 g cider vinegar or lemon juice

Put the water in a stainless steel saucepan. Add the henna powder a little at a time, stirring until the mixture is creamy, with no lumps.

•

Simmer gently for 2–3 minutes, stirring constantly.

•

When lukewarm, distribute over the hair and scalp, using the fingers or a flat paintbrush. It can be put on to dry hair, but if the hair is very oily, it is better to wash it and pat out excess water with a towel first.

•

As the mixture only works when it is wet, you should cover your head with a plastic shower cap, to stop the water evaporating.

•

Sit quietly and let the henna work for at least an hour. Then rinse under lukewarm, running water, removing as much powder as you can.

•

You can follow this up with a mild shampoo, in which case add a tablespoon of cider vinegar, or the freshly squeezed and strained juice of a lemon per quart/liter of water to the final rinse.

•

For badly-damaged hair, serious dandruff or very greasy hair, you can leave the henna on for several hours or even overnight. (Fix the cap well with the aid of clips or a towel around your head.)

# Soapwort shampoo

*This shampoo is particularly good for oily hair with or without dandruff.*

## INGREDIENTS

1 oz/30 g soapwort root (also known as Bouncing Bet)

12½ oz/350 g still mineral water

½ tsp/4 g coarse cooking salt

4 tsp/20 g castor oil

a few drops of essential oil of lavender

4 tsp/20 g herb vinegar

Simmer the finely-chopped root with the water for 20 minutes in a stainless steel pan.

•

Remove from heat and let stand, covered, until tepid. Then, strain into a bottle through a fine sieve. Add the salt and shake the bottle until it dissolves; add the castor oil and essential oil of lavender.

•

Shake well before use. Use as a normal shampoo, diluted with water.

•

It cleans the hair well, even though it has very little lather, and, more importantly, it is not harsh. If you wish, you can wash a second time, after rinsing thoroughly.

•

Add some herb vinegar to the final rinse water: 4 teaspoons per quart/liter of water is sufficient. This will make the hair soft and shiny, more so than a conditioner.

•

Soapwort shampoo keeps for about a week in the refrigerator, or you can store it in an airtight container in the freezer.

•

If you add 2 oz/50 g alcohol – e.g. vodka or brandy – it will keep for much longer.

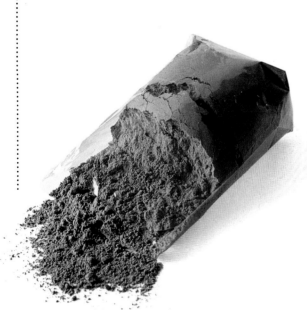

# Clay and herb shampoo

*This unusual way of washing the hair with a type of mud is good for those with oily hair, as it helps normalize sebaceous secretions.*

### INGREDIENTS

2 oz/50 g green airfloat clay or rhassoul mud

2¾ oz/75 g still mineral water

1 tbsp/2 g each of rosemary, sage and thyme leaves, lavender, and nettle flowers

4 tsp/20 g cider vinegar or lemon juice

Prepare the shampoo as described opposite and leave on the hair for 5–10 minutes. Rinse off thoroughly. Add 4 teaspoons of cider vinegar or the freshly squeezed juice of a lemon per quart/liter of water to the final rinse.
•
You can use either green or red airfloat clay or rhassoul mud, a North African clay which is specifically used for washing the hair.

Quantities of clay and water can be adjusted to suit the hair length.
•
If this shampoo dries out your hair, make a mixture of three parts sweet almond oil to one part castor oil. With the tip of a finger, moisten the bristletips of a soft brush with the mixture. Brush the hair with it to soften it and bring it back to life.

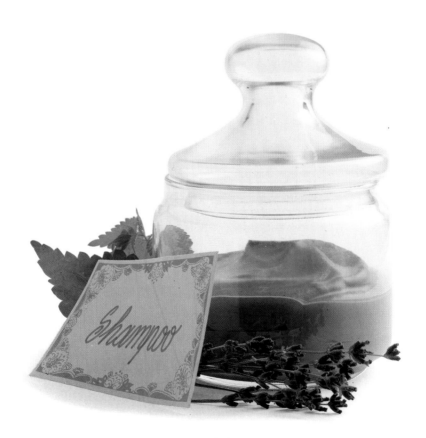

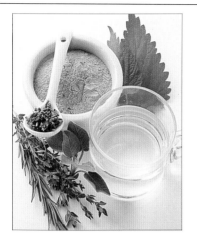

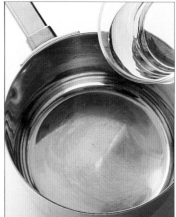

*Prepare the ingredients, weighing the fresh herbs carefully.*

•

*Boil the mineral water.*

•

*Add the herbs, remove from heat immediately and cover.*

•

*Strain after about 15 minutes; add the liquid from the infusion to the clay and mix thoroughly.*

•

*Massage into the scalp.*

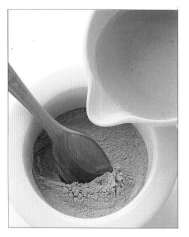

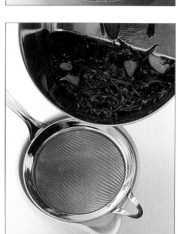

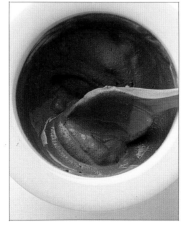

# Panama wood shampoo

*In places where Panama wood is indigenous (Central and South America) this shampoo is used to promote hair growth.*

## INGREDIENTS

1 oz/30 g fragments of Panama wood bark

14 oz/400 g still mineral water

¹⁄₃ oz/10 g rosemary leaves

4 tsp/20 g castor oil

4 tsp/20 g herb vinegar

Put the bark and water into a stainless steel saucepan and leave to soak overnight.

•

Simmer for 20 minutes. Turn off the heat and add the rosemary leaves, which must not boil, or their highly-volatile essential oil will evaporate.

•

Leave to infuse until lukewarm, then strain into a bottle and add the castor oil.

•

Shake well before use.

•

Use as a dilute shampoo, wetting the hair with it. Massage into the scalp with the fingertips and leave for a few minutes.

•

Rinse thoroughly under running water.

•

Add a tablespoon of herb vinegar per quart/liter of water to the final rinse. This will add luster to the hair and revitalize it.

# Emollient scalp treatment

*This treatment makes dull, lifeless hair soft and lustrous, and has an anti-inflammatory action on the scalp, helping to control dandruff and itchiness.*

## INGREDIENTS

1 tsp/5 g sweet almond oil

½ tsp/2 g avocado oil

½ tsp/2 g castor oil

15 drops essential oil of rosemary or lavender

1 egg yolk

4 tsp/20 g liquid honey

4 tsp/20 g cider vinegar or lemon juice

Mix the oils in a cup and gently massage into the hair and scalp. Cover the head with an old towel and leave for 15–30 minutes.

•

A short oil treatment before shampooing makes the shampoo more effective. It softens clogged pores and dandruff scales, and helps counteract the drying action of commercial shampoos.

•

Even better results are achieved by adding egg yolk and honey to the oils. Mix them together thoroughly in a cup. Spread the mixture all over the hair and scalp and cover with a towel or shower cap.

•

If the mixture drips or there is some left over, spread it over the face and neck – it makes a nourishing face mask.

Leave for at least half an hour, then rinse off with tepid water and shampoo the hair as usual.

•

Add 4 teaspoons of cider vinegar or fresh lemon juice per quart/liter of water to the final rinse.

•

The quantities can be varied proportionally, to suit the length of hair being treated.

# White wine and Panama wood shampoo

*This shampoo combines the stimulating effects of Panama
wood and white wine with the emollient properties of the oils;
it also helps control dandruff.*

### INGREDIENTS

2 oz/50 g finely-chopped or powdered
Panama wood bark

14¼ oz/400 g dry white wine

1½ oz/40 g 95° proof alcohol

1 tsp/5 g castor oil

1 tsp/5 g avocado oil

a few drops/3 g essential oil of
rosemary

Using a wide-mouthed jar with an
airtight lid, steep the bark in the
wine and alcohol for a week,
shaking occasionally.
•

Pour into a bottle, first through a
sieve and then through a paper
filter. Add the oils.
•

Shake before use and apply the
shampoo to wet hair, massaging
gently. Leave on for a few minutes.
Rinse thoroughly under running
water.
•

This shampoo will keep for quite a
long time, even at room
temperature.

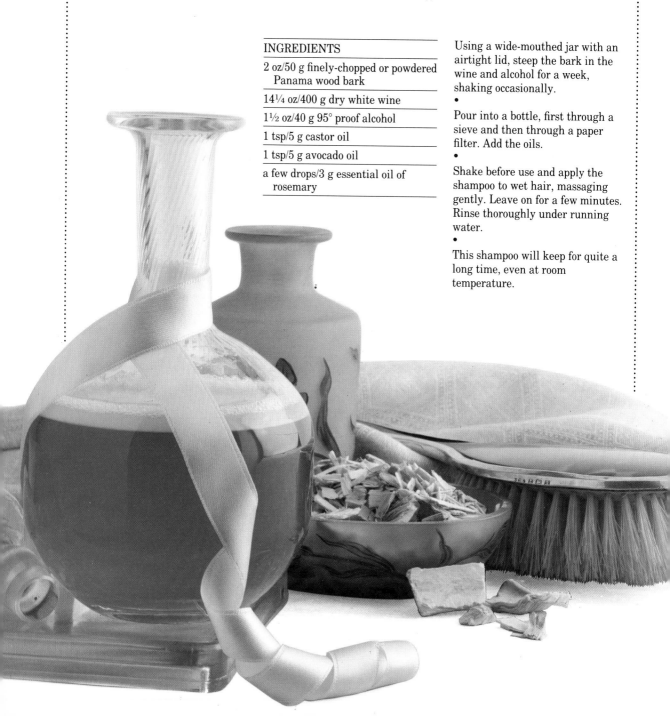

# Vegetable protein shampoo

*Many old recipes for shampoo use puréed chickpeas, lentils, peas, beans, etc. They are particularly good for brittle and damaged hair.*

## INGREDIENTS

2 oz/50 g very finely-milled flour of any type of pulse

14¼ oz/400 g still mineral water

4 tsp/20 g herb vinegar or lemon juice

Put the flour into a stainless steel saucepan. Add the water a little at a time and mix thoroughly.

•

You can save time by using a blender or food processor which will make a smoother mixture.

•

Cook over a very low heat for at least 20 minutes, stirring constantly. Make sure the mixture does not stick to the bottom of the pan.

•

Remove from heat, and let cool. When lukewarm, apply the mixture to wet hair, massaging it carefully and slowly into the scalp. Use generously.

Rinse thoroughly under lukewarm running water. The success of the shampoo depends on your removing every trace of the mixture.

•

Add 4 teaspoons of herb vinegar or lemon juice per quart/liter of water to the final rinsing water.

•

It is important that the flour is very finely milled, without any trace of husk.

•

If you cannot find finely-milled pulse flour to buy, you can make your own out of dried peas or beans. (Make sure they have no skins.) Soak the dried peas or beans overnight, cook until soft, and then sieve or put into a blender (30 seconds at low speed and 30 seconds at high speed). Only the soft pulp should be used.

•

This shampoo keeps for a couple of days in the refrigerator, or it can be frozen in an airtight container.

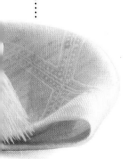

# Dry shampoo

*This is a dry shampoo for those who for one reason or another cannot use water on their hair. It is most effective on shorter hair.*

## INGREDIENTS

5 oz/150 g coarsely-milled maize or corn flour

30 drops essential oil of lemon

20 drops castor oil

Mix the ingredients in a blender for a few seconds.

•

Spread a large towel over a table, sit down and bend the head forward. Distribute pinches of the mixture over the hair and scalp, and massage them in very gently.

•

Take care to massage the whole head slowly and methodically, dividing it into sections and working on one area at a time.

•

With the head still bent forward, comb and then brush out the meal. Continue brushing and combing until the hair is shiny and free of all traces of the shampoo.

•

It is important to use coarsely-milled flour; semolina or couscous are also suitable.

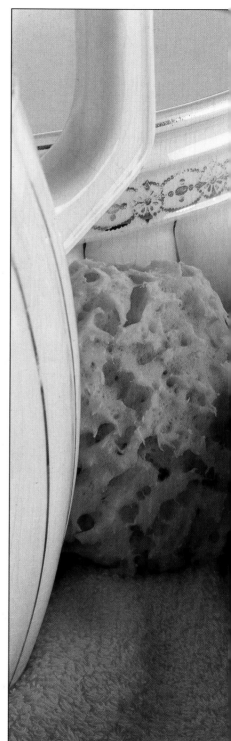

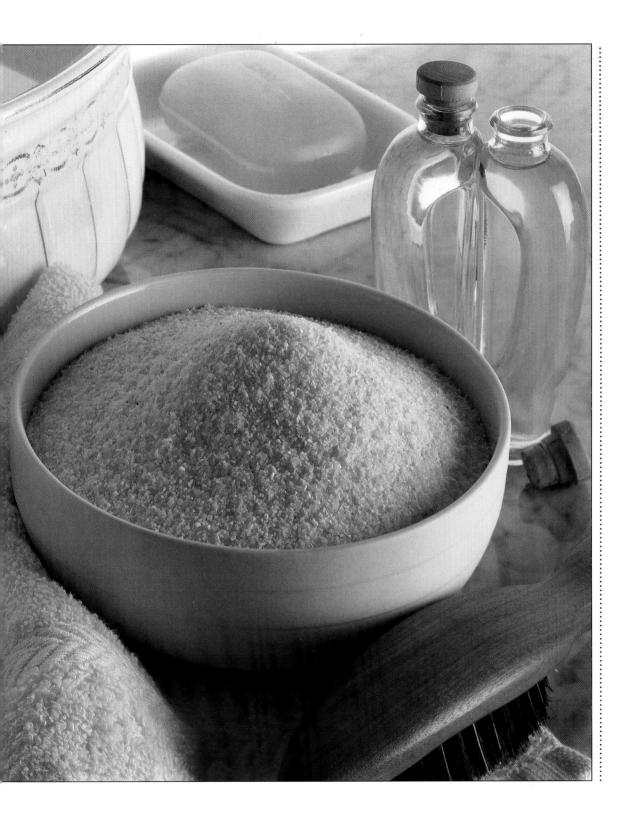

# Egg shampoo

*This is one of the oldest methods of cleaning the hair, and still one of the most effective.*

## INGREDIENTS

1 or 2 fresh eggs

2–3½ oz/50–100 g still mineral water

1 tbsp/15 g cider vinegar or lemon juice

The eggs should be removed from the refrigerator at least an hour before they are needed and the water should be approximately body temperature (98°F/37°C).
•
Mix the ingredients in a blender for 30 seconds at low speed.
•
Wet your hair and massage the mixture slowly and systematically into the scalp.
•
The success of the shampoo depends on a long massage and an even longer rinse under lukewarm water (if the water is any hotter than that, the egg will begin to set!). Continue rinsing out until all traces of egg have disappeared.

Add a tablespoon of cider vinegar or freshly-squeezed lemon juice per quart/liter of water to the final rinse.
•
The hair will be clean, shiny, light and airy.
•
This mixture does not keep and should be used immediately.

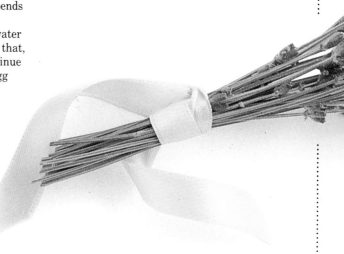

# Nettle hair lotion

*Nettles form the basis of many folk remedies, and their benefits to hair have long been recognized. Nettle recipes have a stimulating and therapeutic effect.*

## INGREDIENTS

3½ oz/100g fresh nettles, complete with roots

⅓ oz/10 g broken bay leaves

7 oz/200 g 95° proof liqueur alcohol

4 tsp/20 g castor oil

2 tsp/10 g wheatgerm oil

1 tsp/5 g essential oil of lavender

1½ pints/¾ liter still mineral water or cider vinegar

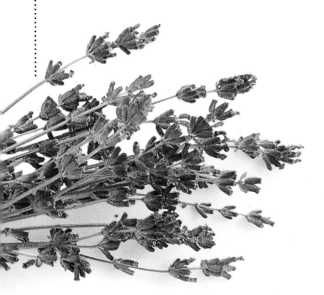

Protecting your hands with rubber gloves, wash the nettles under running water. Make sure that all the soil has been washed off the roots.

•

Cut the nettles into small pieces with stainless steel scissors, directly over the jug of the blender. Add the alcohol. Blend for a minute at low speed and a minute at high speed, until you have a liquid green pulp.

•

Transfer to a wide-mouthed glass jar, add the bay leaves, seal and steep for 13 days, shaking occasionally. Strain the mixture through a fine sieve and then a paper filter, squeezing out the pulp. Pour into a bottle and add the water or cider vinegar, castor oil, wheatgerm oil and oil of lavender.

•

Shake well before use. Between hair washes rub the lotion into the scalp using a piece of cotton wool/cotton. It will help prevent oily hair and dandruff. You can also use it before or after shampooing. Before shampooing, massage into the hair and scalp and leave for 10–15 minutes. If used after shampooing, add a tablespoon per quart/liter of water to the final rinse. The lotion can be stored at room temperature.

# Cider vinegar conditioning rinse

*This rinse makes the hair soft and shiny and easy to comb. It is also useful as an anti-dandruff lotion between shampoos.*

## INGREDIENTS

1 pint/5½ liter cider vinegar

1 oz/25 g fresh nettles (use the whole plant)

⅔ oz/20 g chopped ivy leaves

⅓ oz/10 g walnut leaves

⅓ oz/10 g sage leaves

⅓ oz/10 g rosemary leaves

⅓ oz/10 g thyme leaves

2 oz/50 g 95° proof liqueur alcohol

2 tsp/10 g castor oil

This treatment is especially recommended for brown hair as it brings out the natural highlights.
•

Remember that aromatic vinegars tend to go cloudy and form sediments, but this does not alter their properties.
•

Prepare the lotion as shown opposite and shake before use. You can use it immediately after shampooing, adding a tablespoon per quart/liter of water to the final rinse, or you can massage small amounts into the scalp with a piece of cotton wool/cotton between hair washes.
•

This is a good treatment for dandruff and itchy scalp as it acts as an antiseptic against the bacteria which multiply on dandruff, especially on oily hair.
•

It will keep for a long time at room temperature.

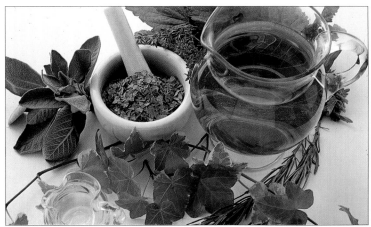

Steep the herbs in the vinegar and alcohol for two weeks in a wide-mouthed, airtight jar, shaking the jar occasionally.

•

The nettles must be well washed, especially the roots, and then patted dry with a towel and finely chopped with a sharp blade or in a blender.

•

You can use ivy leaves straight from the garden, in which case you should add another ⅓ oz/10 g washed, dried and chopped like the nettles.

•

Strain the liquid from the chopped herbs into a bottle, first through a sieve and then through a paper filter. Add the oil.

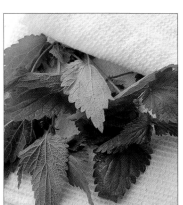

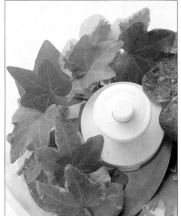

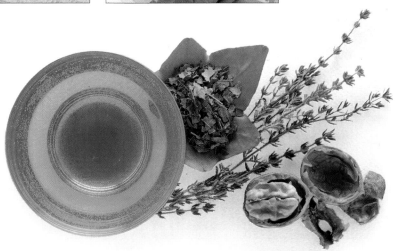

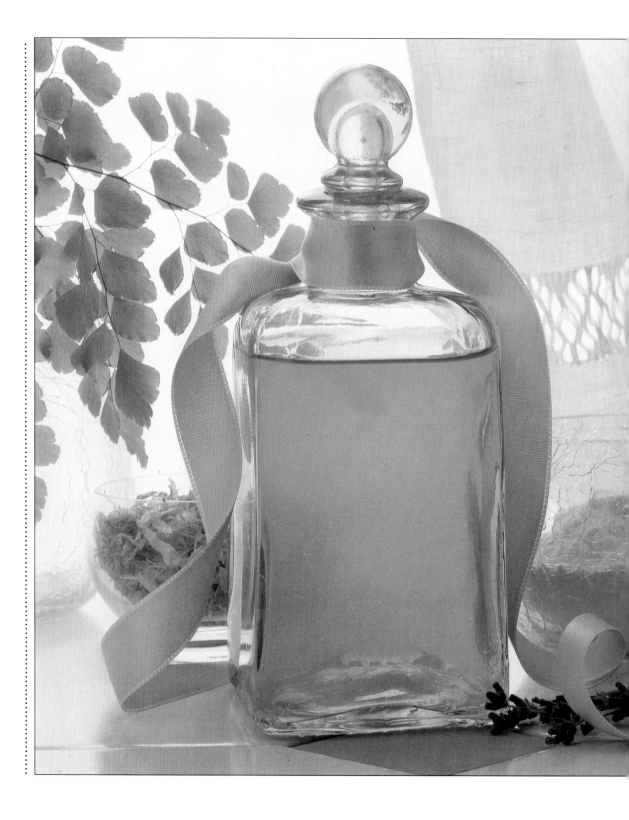

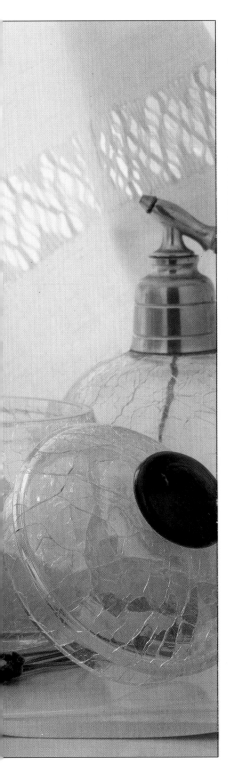

# Lemon conditioner

*This brings out the highlights in fair hair, and makes all hair soft and manageable.*

## INGREDIENTS

2 lemons

⅔ oz/20 g marigold flowers

⅔ oz/20 g chamomile flowers

1–1¼ oz/30 g finely chopped or powdered rhubarb root

2 oz/50 g acacia honey

1 pint/½ liter cider vinegar

2 oz/50 g 95° proof liqueur alcohol

Put the vinegar and rhubarb into a stainless steel saucepan. Bring to a boil and simmer very gently for 10 minutes.

•

Add the chamomile, marigold and zest of the two lemons; cover the pan and simmer for another 5 minutes. Remove from heat.

•

Let stand covered until tepid. Filter through a fine sieve into a bottle. Make sure you squeeze out any liquid in the herbs left in the sieve.

•

Add the honey, alcohol and squeezed and strained lemon juice.

•

Use it diluted after shampooing, adding a tablespoon per quart/liter of water to the final rinse. For stronger highlights, apply the mixture neat and leave on for at least half an hour, covering the head with a shower cap.

•

Take care because, in undiluted form, this liquid will dye any materials it comes into contact with.

•

It will keep for quite a long time at room temperature.

# Chamomile and marigold oil

*This mixture protects the skin of young and old alike. As a pre-shampoo treatment, it acts as an emollient and brings out highlights in fair hair.*

## INGREDIENTS

1¼ oz/30 g dried chamomile flowers

1¼ oz/30 g dried marigold flowers, chopped

10 oz/275 g sweet almond oil

1 oz/25 g wheatgerm oil

Steep the flowers in the oils in a wide-mouthed, airtight jar. Leave it in the sun for at least a month. Choose a jar of the right size, as there should be as little air space as possible between the surface of the oil and the lid to limit oxidization.

•

If preparing the mixture in winter, you can use a gentle source of heat. For example, stand it near (not on!) a radiator or in the warm draft of air behind a refrigerator.

•

After the maceration process is complete, pour the mixture through a strainer into a bottle. Press all the liquid out of the plant material with a potato masher.

•

Use the liquid as an occasional pre-shampoo treatment for any type of scalp irritation, such as pruritus (itchy scalp), redness or dandruff, whether the hair is dry or oily. It will also bring out the highlights in fair or light brown hair.

•

It keeps for a long time in small, well-filled and sealed dark glass bottles.

# Bay oil

*This is a good oily, pre-shampoo treatment for dark hair. It helps protect the colour and sheen of the hair as the years go by.*

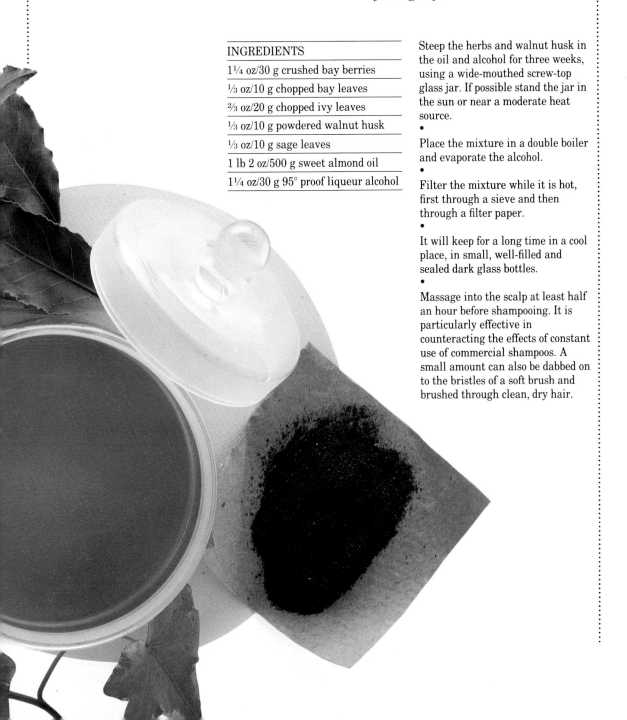

## INGREDIENTS

| | |
|---|---|
| 1¼ oz/30 g crushed bay berries |
| ⅓ oz/10 g chopped bay leaves |
| ⅔ oz/20 g chopped ivy leaves |
| ⅓ oz/10 g powdered walnut husk |
| ⅓ oz/10 g sage leaves |
| 1 lb 2 oz/500 g sweet almond oil |
| 1¼ oz/30 g 95° proof liqueur alcohol |

Steep the herbs and walnut husk in the oil and alcohol for three weeks, using a wide-mouthed screw-top glass jar. If possible stand the jar in the sun or near a moderate heat source.

•

Place the mixture in a double boiler and evaporate the alcohol.

•

Filter the mixture while it is hot, first through a sieve and then through a filter paper.

•

It will keep for a long time in a cool place, in small, well-filled and sealed dark glass bottles.

•

Massage into the scalp at least half an hour before shampooing. It is particularly effective in counteracting the effects of constant use of commercial shampoos. A small amount can also be dabbed on to the bristles of a soft brush and brushed through clean, dry hair.

# Cider vinegar with herbs

*This lotion helps alleviate many scalp disorders – dandruff, pruritus or itchy scalp, and various types of irritation – and it complements the action of natural shampoos.*

## INGREDIENTS

10½ oz/300 g cider vinegar

⅔ oz/20 g marigold mother tincture

⅓ oz/10 g nettle mother tincture

1 oz/30 g propolis mother tincture

2 tsp/10 g sage mother tincture

2 tsp/10 g avocado oil

Mix the ingredients together. Shake before use. Rub the vinegar into the hair and scalp between hair washes.

•

If you massage the scalp daily with pieces of cotton wool/cotton soaked in the mixture, you will find that you need to shampoo less often. Store at room temperature.

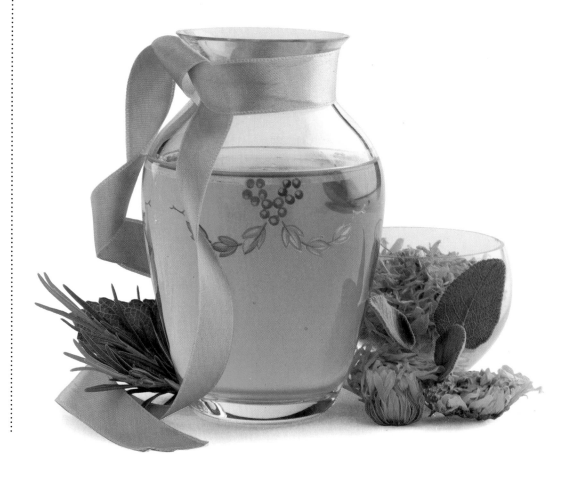

# HENNA

Henna is a harmless vegetable dye, used for thousands of years in India, the Middle East and North Africa to dye the hair, beard, eyebrows, nails, palms and soles various shades of red. Henna comes in the form of a greenish powder, made from dried leaves of Lawsonia inermis. Mixed with boiling water into a thin, creamy solution, it is applied to the hair, and left to take effect, preferably in a warm place.

When using henna on your hair, it is impossible to predict the final results, so you need to test it on a sample of hair. The easiest way is to use the strands left on your comb each day. There are five factors to take into consideration before using henna:

– The colour of your hair. You may get yellow, copper or titian red overtones – although never lighter than your hair. White hair may turn bright orange but harmless vegetable dyes including walnut husk, indigo, alkanet can be added to tone down the colour. If the treatment is repeated periodically, the results will be better and the colour more penetrating, even on white or grey hair which require repeated applications to achieve natural-looking results. If you start using henna at the first signs of grey hair, and repeat the process each time the roots become visible, you will not notice the gradual change over the years.

– Your hair type. Some hair absorbs colour easily; others are more resistant.

– The type of henna used. Like all natural products, henna varies according to the country in which it is grown. For instance, Iranian henna is slightly different from Egyptian. Even the regional and climatic variations within one country can affect its properties.

– The amount of time it is left on the hair. The longer it is left, the stronger the colour will be.

– Any other herbs which are added.

Henna treatments are certainly longer and more complicated than chemical dyes. But your efforts will be well rewarded: the product is harmless, and the results will be better. Henna produces a wide range of subtle colour; makes the hair more resilient; adds body; and is good for the scalp, which will be less oily and produce less dandruff.

# HIGHLIGHTS

A decoction of one or more plants from the list on page 53 will add highlights to the hair if used as an after-shampoo rinse, even without the henna. The results will not last long, however, if the treatment is not repeated. As in the case of henna, these herbal rinses add highlights to your hair but do not cover up the original colour. Amounts suggested can be varied depending on the results you get from testing them on your own hair. You can also vary the time the herbs are boiled – from 5 to 30 minutes. Obviously the longer you boil them, the stronger the colours will be, although you will have to use more water to allow for evaporation.

If you need to add 95° proof alcohol to the decoction, then wait until it has cooled to lukewarm, then let stand, covered, for a few hours before straining it.

If you use light-coloured rinses (from gold to yellow and ocher) you could emulate the fashionable ladies of a bygone age, and dry your hair in the sun.

For more lasting results, make a creamy compress made by mixing the powder of one or more herbs with boiling water, as with the henna. Spread this over clean, damp hair and leave on for half an hour to an hour.

# Henna rinse

*This gives brown hair beautiful copper highlights and is an excellent conditioner.*

### INGREDIENTS

2 oz/50 g red henna

12½ oz/350 g still mineral water

4 tsp/20 g cider vinegar or the juice of half a lemon

Using a stainless steel saucepan, boil the water and add the henna powder a little at a time, stirring constantly until it has the consistency of cream or butter.

•

Add the cider vinegar or lemon juice, which helps the henna to work. Some people prefer to use overripe yogurt as an acidifier.

•

In some Middle Eastern countries, henna powder is dissolved in yogurt the night before use: apart from strengthening the colour, it makes the mixture creamier.

•

The hair should be washed and towel-dried, so that it is damp, but not wet. Add some aromatic vinegar to the final rinsing water.

•

Draw partings on the head to ensure that you distribute the henna evenly, and apply the mixture with a flat paintbrush, using disposable gloves to avoid staining your hands.

If you plan to leave it for several hours, smear vaseline on the forehead at the hairline to prevent the colour from running.

•

Cover your hair with a shower cap to keep it moist.

•

Heat speeds up the process. Put an old woollen hat over the shower cap or in the summer, sit in the sun. Some people cover their heads with tin foil which is another good insulator, while others use a hairdryer.

•

If you experiment with a lock of hair first, it will give you some idea of how long to leave the mixture on; it could be anything from half an hour to three hours.

•

Rinse your hair very thoroughly under lukewarm water to remove all traces of mixture. The best way to do this is to use the shower head in the bath, holding it with one hand and massaging the hair and scalp gently with the other.

# HENNA WITH OTHER HERBS

*As already mentioned, henna can exhibit a wide range of hues, depending on the colour of your hair, your hair type, the quality of the henna, which varies according to where it comes from, and the length of time it is left on the hair.*

*You can extend the range of tints by combining it with other vegetable dyes. Instead of using boiling water, use strong tea or coffee to tone down the red. Similar results can be obtained by using decoctions of walnut husk or artichoke leaves. Use at least three tablespoons in 14¼ oz/400 g of still mineral water: simmer for 15 minutes, strain and dissolve the henna in the liquid. You can soften or intensify the colours by halving or doubling the amount of herbs. If you want even stronger colours, add the plants in the table or others to the henna in powdered form. They should be available from herbalists.*

*Henna acts as a fixative, not only for its own colour, but for any others with which it is combined. Therefore at least ⅓ of the mixture should consist of henna. The table lists a number of plants which are used as vegetable dyes and can be bought in powdered form and added to the henna, or made into a decoction, into which the henna should be dissolved.*

| Plant | Part used | Average dose per 3½ oz/100 g water | Colour | Remarks |
|---|---|---|---|---|
| Roman Chamomile | flowers | 1 oz/25 g | honey highlights | used on its own, the effects are not permanent |
| German Chamomile | flowers | 1 oz/25 g | honey highlights | best combined with rhubarb, tea, saffron |
| Safflower | flowers | 1 oz/25 g | orange-yellow | used in combination with saffron |
| Turmeric | root | ⅔ oz/20 g | yellow | stronger with 20% alcohol |
| Rhubarb | root | ⅓–⅔ oz/10–20 g | golden yellow | fixative in mixtures with saffron and chamomile |
| Saffron | stigmata | 1–2 g | yellow | with walnut, reddish; with black tea, golden |
| Annatto | seeds | ⅓ oz/10 g | red | soluble in oil |
| Henna | leaves | ½ oz/15 g | orange-red | |
| Java jute | flowers | ⅔ oz/20 g | reddish | |
| Alkanet | root | ½ oz/15 g | red-brown | |
| Madder | root | ⅓–⅔ oz/10–20 g | red | best if you add 20% alcohol |
| Quebracho | wood and bark | ¼ oz/10 g | dark red | combined with henna products, brownish red shades |
| Catechu | dry extract from wood | ¼ oz/5–10 g | reddish brown | gives chestnut tint to henna |
| Logwood | wood | ½ oz/15 g | yellowish red-brown violet | in acid solution in neutral solution in alkaline solution |
| Ivy | leaves | ⅓–½ oz/10–15 g | brown | with henna, gives chestnut tints |
| Indigo | leaves | ⅓–½ oz/10–15 g | blue-black | with walnut, darker chestnut results from using henna |
| Walnut | leaves | ⅓–½ oz/10–15 g | brown | with 25–50% henna gives beautiful chestnut shades |
| | husk | ½–⅔ oz/15–20 g | dark brown | |
| Gall nut | the gall | ⅓–1 oz/10–25 g | brown | best if you add 20% alcohol |
| Sandalwood | wood | ⅔–1 oz/20–30 g | reddish brown | smells good |
| Black tea leaves | | ⅓–½ oz/10–15 g | brown | acts as a fixative |
| Artichoke leaves | | ⅔ oz/20 g | brown | |

# Henna with oil

*Henna tends to dry the hair out, so some may prefer this treatment.*

INGREDIENTS

2 oz/50 g red henna

12½ oz/350 g still mineral water

4 tsp/20 g sweet almond oil

You may prefer to use other types of oil, either alone or in combination. A good mixture consists of:
2 tbsp/30 g sweet almond oil
2 tbsp/30 g avocado oil
2 tbsp/30 g wheatgerm oil
1 tbsp/15 g castor oil

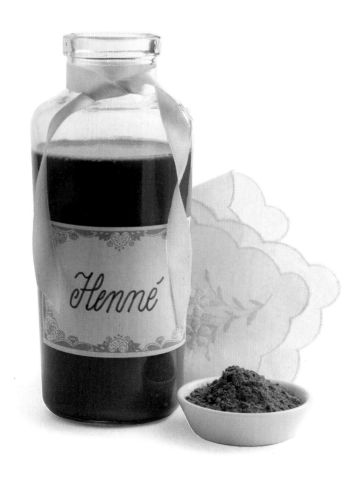

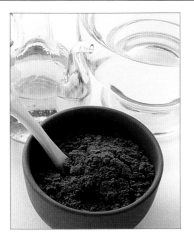

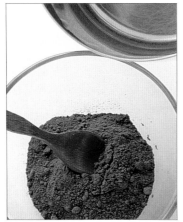

Boil the water and dissolve the henna in it, adding a little at a time until smooth.

Add the oil, stirring until it is thoroughly amalgamated.

Protecting your hands with gloves, apply the mixture to freshly washed, towel-dried hair, using a flat paintbrush.

Treat as for plain henna, covering the head with a shower cap to retain heat and moisture.

Rinse under hot running water. You will need to spend even longer rinsing than you would for a plain henna treatment.

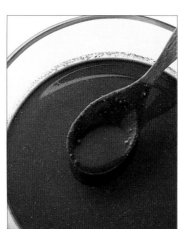

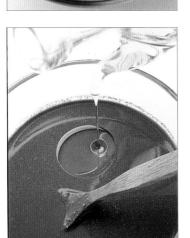

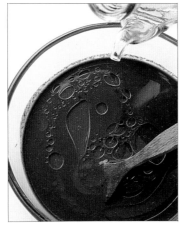

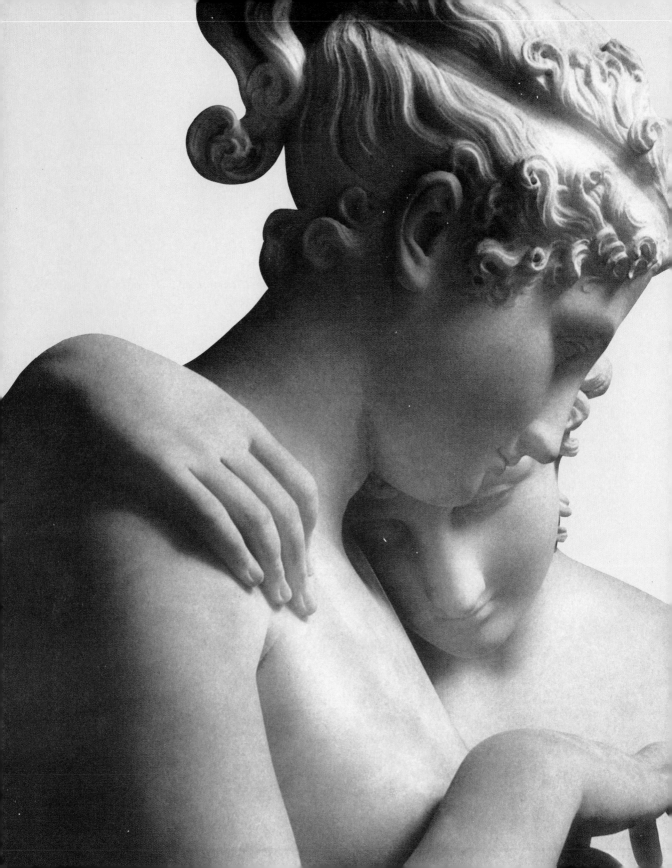

# The face

*What modern dermatology has added to the
ancient teachings of the art of cosmetics is the
simple rule that any substance to be applied to the
skin must follow the basic laws of hygiene. This
means any product that may be toxic or in any way
imperfect should be avoided. Or, in other words,
anything that is fit to eat can be applied safely to
the skin. This chapter includes recipes for
cleansing milks, toners, creams and face masks
that are made from items you normally buy when
you are shopping for groceries.*

When washing the face, cleansing milk is better than soap. Although soap is good for removing dirt, and feels fresh and clean, it often cleans the skin too thoroughly, and can upset the fine hydro-lipid (water-oil) balance on which a good complexion depends. This is also the case with commercial shampoos and bubble baths. Cleansing milk on the other hand, is generally in the form of an emulsion, a type of "mayonnaise" made of oil and water. This works better than soap, because the oil dissolves the thickest grease on the skin, without stripping it away completely. Water completes the process by dissolving dust and water-soluble salts, which are left on the skin by perspiration. If you then rinse your face thoroughly, your skin will be clean, but not dried out. This method would be ideal if cleansing milk was made as it was four hundred years ago, by pounding almonds and rose water in a mortar for hours. Today's cleansing milks often use petrochemicals like vaseline and paraffin oil instead of vegetable oils, which are kinder to the skin. Even those which are based on vegetable oils contain antioxidants, antifungal agents and preservatives to stop the oil from going rancid, and these can trigger allergic reactions. The table on page 59 lists some of the edible substances which have been used on the skin as an alternative to soap in the past, either on their own or in combinations. They are often better than soap, particularly for people with sensitive skin.

You should make your cleansing milk using ingredients in the table that work for your skin type. The milk should then be used only by you. Bear this in mind when considering quantities as well as ingredients. Recipes will vary depending on the season, your lifestyle, and the type of make-up you use. However, you should choose one or more substances from each group, and the final product should have a creamy-liquid consistency.

Some substances can be used on their own, particularly for cleansing very sensitive skin, to which no make-up has been applied. For example, milk, yogurt, ricotta cheese, cream and butter; maple syrup, molasses, malt, honey, and other sugary syrups; oils and oily substances; the pulp of many fruits (avocado, apple, banana) and some vegetables, either raw or cooked (potatoes and carrots); refined cereal and legume flours and starches, either mixed to a paste with water, or cooked for a few minutes over a low heat, stirring constantly with a wooden spoon; and white wine. Fragrance (essential oils) should not be added if you are prone to allergies or before sunbathing, as some of them are photosensitive and can cause permanent discoloration of the skin.

Most of the ingredients should be familiar to anyone with basic culinary skills, and cooking experience is enough to tell you which combinations are appropriate and what the final consistency will be. Any mistakes you make will be harmless, and inexpensive, given

that the amounts used are quite small. Follow your instincts in choosing the ingredients, as each of us has affinities for or individual reactions to certain products. The important thing is to approach the subject with an open mind. After a few experiments the results will spur you on. The tables on the next few pages will provide you with enough information to choose those ingredients best suited to you. Examples 1–6 on page 60 will show you how to begin. Further on in the book, you will find several recipes based on ancient cleansers which have been modernized.

All solutions should be mixed thoroughly, ideally in a blender for a minute at low speed and a minute at high speed. For the last two recipes (on page 60), you will need a press or juice extractor to obtain the cabbage juice and lily bulb juice. If you do not have a food processor with this accessory, it is worth borrowing a friend's because cabbage juice is extremely good in a face pack as a treatment for acne, and the thick juice of the lily bulb makes a very good skin smoothener and anti-wrinkle treatment.

Sprouts (example 4) are mainly composed of tissues in a rapid state of growth, full of active principles and valuable eaten or applied externally.

Nearly all types of seeds can be germinated in a propagator or by soaking them on a plate covered with another, upside down like a clam. Rinse the seeds twice daily, they will start to germinate after two or three days, then drain the water off the seeds to stop them from

## INGREDIENTS FOR CLEANSING MILKS

### Proteinaceous binding agents
Whole eggs, egg  white, egg yolk, animal gelatin, milk,
yogurt, ricotta cheese

■

### Sugar binding agents
Sugar, sugar-cane molasses, sugar-beet molasses, barley
malt, rice malt, maple syrup, honey

■

### Oils and fats
Sweet almond oil, wheatgerm oil, extra-virgin olive oil, soya
oil, corn oil, sunflower oil, avocado oil, jojoba oil, evening
primrose oil, coconut oil, cocoa butter, cream, butter

■

### Vegetable matter
Fruit, vegetables and herbs (see page 61)

■

### Thickeners, emollients, emulsifiers
Rice starch, wheat starch, cornflour (cornstarch), potato
starch,
cereal flours (wheat, barley, oat, rye, millet),
legume flours (peas, beans, lentils, chickpeas, soya beans,
lupin seeds, fenugreek)
agar agar, clays (white, red, green)
sweet almond flour, powdered orris root, soya lecithin

■

### Extracts and miscellaneous
buds macerated in glycerine (MG)*
mother tinctures (MT),*
oily substances, royal jelly, white wine, wine vinegar, cider
vinegar, yeast, propolis, beeswax, beer

■

### Perfumes
Essential oils (EO)*

* Note that the recipes in the following chapters will make repeated use of
these abbreviations.

going mouldy. The sprouts
should be used whole, when they
are about 1 in (2–3 cm) long. As
soon as the leaves appear,
remove the top dish. The plants
will have more active principles
if they are exposed to the light.
At this point, rinse them three
times a day. The mixtures, like
dishes made with them, will
keep for a day or two in the
refrigerator, but are best used
immediately.

## EXAMPLES OF CLEANSING MILKS

|  | HEAVY MAKE-UP |  | LIGHT MAKE-UP OR NO MAKE-UP |
|---|---|---|---|
| **1** | Combination skin, with poor tone | **2** | Dry, fair, sensitive skin |
| **Binding agent** | 1 egg white | | 1 egg white |
| **Oils and greases** | 4 tsp/20 g cream<br>2 tsp/10 g almond oil | | 1 tsp/4 g avocado oil<br>1 tsp/4 g jojoba oil<br>1 tsp/4 g wheatgerm oil |
| **Vegetable matter** | 2¼ oz/60 g banana flesh | | 2 oz/60 g cucumber flesh |
| **Thickeners emollients emulsifiers** | ⅕ oz/5 g potato flour<br>⅕ oz/5 g chickpea flour | | 2 tsp/10 g fine rice flour |
| **Extracts** | 20 drops poplar bud MG<br>10 drops sage MT | | 30 drops lime/linden MG |
| **Perfumes** | 5 drops rosemary EO | | 5 drops lemon EO |
| **3** | Oily, inflamed, blotchy skin | **4** | Oily, inflamed, ageing skin with lines |
| **Binding agent** | 1 egg yolk<br>2 tsp/10 g acacia honey | | 1 egg yolk<br>2 tsp/10 g sugar-cane molasses |
| **Oils and greases** | 1½ tsp/8 g sweet almond oil<br>1½ tsp/8 g castor oil | | 1 tsp/4 g wheatgerm oil<br>1 tsp/4 g jojoba oil |
| **Vegetable matter** | 2 oz/50 g tomato flesh | | 1¼ oz/30 g watercress sprouts<br>⅔ oz/20 g fenugreek sprouts |
| **Thickeners emollients emulsifiers** | ⅓ oz/10 g chickpea flour<br>1 oz/30 g white clay | | 1¼ oz/30 g fenugreek powder |
| **Extracts** | 1 tsp/4 g marigold oil<br>1 tsp/4 g chamomile oil<br>30 drops St. John's wort MT | | 2 tsp/10 g rosemary oil<br>30 drops ginseng MT<br>20 drops hop MT |
| **Perfumes** | 5 drops yarrow EO | | 5 drops rosemary EO |
| **5** | Oily skin with acne and open pores | **6** | Dry, sensitive skin, with premature wrinkles |
| **Binding agent** | 2 oz/50 g ricotta cheese | | 2 oz/50 g ricotta cheese |
| **Oils and greases** | 2 tsp/10 g avocado oil<br>2 tsp/10 g sweet almond oil<br>2 tsp/10 g extra-virgin olive oil | | 2 tsp/10 g avocado oil<br>2 tsp/10 g wheatgerm oil<br>1 tsp/5 g jojoba oil |
| **Vegetable matter** | 2 oz/50 g cabbage juice | | 2 oz/50 g fresh madonna lily bulb |
| **Thickeners emollients emulsifiers** | ¾ oz/20 g brewer's yeast<br>1½ oz/40 g orris root powder | | 1 tsp/5 g white clay |
| **Extracts** | 30 drops witch hazel MT | | 30 drops rosemary MT<br>10 drops fenugreek MT<br>10 drops hop MT |
| **Perfumes** | 3 drops thyme EO | | 5 drops orange EO |

# THE MAIN PROPERTIES OF FRUIT, VEGETABLES AND HERBS

| Emollient and anti-inflammatory | Astringent | Antiseptic and balsamic | Tonic and firming |
|---|---|---|---|
| Almond *fruit* | Benzoin *resin or gum* | Anise *seeds* | Apple *fruit* |
| Apple *fruit* | Catechu *dried extract* | Basil *leaves* | Apricot *fruit* |
| Avocado *fruit* | Cinchona *bark* | Benzoin *resin* | Avocado *fruit* |
| Banana *fruit* | Cornflower *flower* | Camphor *essential oil* | Beetroot *leaves* |
| Cereal *flour* (oat, wheat, etc.) | Horse-chestnut *seeds or nuts* | Fennel *seeds* | Carrot *root* |
| Cucumber *fruit* | Hypericum (see St. John's wort) | Juniper *leaves* | Chervil *leaves* |
| Elder *flowers* | Honeysuckle *leaves* | Lavender *flowers* | Cider vinegar |
| Everlasting (see Helichrysum) | Ivy *leaves* | Lemon *leaves (peel)* | Cucumber *fruit* |
| Fenugreek *seeds* (powdered) | Lemon *fruit (juice)* | Lemon balm *leaves* | Dandelion *flower* |
| Fig *fruit* | Black poplar *buds* | Lemon verbena *leaves* | Everlasting (see Helichrysum) |
| Flax *seeds* | Madonna lily *bulb* | Licorice *root* | Fenugreek *sprouts* |
| German chamomile *flowers* | Myrrh *resin* | Black poplar *buds* | Helichrysum *flower* |
| Helichrysum *flowers* | Myrtle *leaves* | Marjoram *leaves* | Horse-chestnut *seeds* |
| Honeysuckle *leaves* | Oak *bark* | Myrrh *resin* | Horsetail *stems* |
| Hypericum (see St. John's wort) | Oak *gall* | Orange *flowers (peel)* | Lemon *fruit (juice)* |
| Ivy *leaves* | Orange *fruit (juice)* | Oregano *leaves* | Melilot *flowering heads* |
| Lemon *fruit (juice)* | Pomegranate *fruit* | Peppermint *leaves* | Parsley *leaves* |
| Lemon verbena *leaves* | Red rose *flowers* | Rosemary *leaves* | Peach *fruit* |
| Lettuce *leaves* | St. John's wort *flower heads* | Sage *leaves* | Plum *fruit* |
| Licorice *root* | Silver birch *bark* | Sandalwood *essential oil* | Red currant *fruit* |
| Lime/Linden *flowers with bracts* | Strawberry *fruit* | Silver fir *leaves* | Rosemary *flowers, leaves* |
| Madonna lily *bulb* | Tea *leaves* | Swiss mountain pine *buds* | Sage *leaves* |
| Mallow *flowers and leaves* | Tomato *fruit* | Thyme *leaves* | Silver birch *leaves, buds* |
| Marigold *flowers* | Tormentil *root* | | Strawberry *fruit* |
| Marsh mallow *root* | Walnut *leaves* | | Sweet woodruff *leaves* |
| Musk melon *fruit* | | | Tansy *flower* |
| Orange *flowers* | | | Tea *leaves* |
| Orange *fruit (juice)* | | | Watercress *sprouts* |
| Parsley *leaves* | | | Wheat *sprouts* |
| Pear *fruit* | | | White dead-nettle *flower heads* |
| Plantain *leaves* | | | Yellow gentian *root* |
| Potato *tuber* | | | |
| Psyllium *husks* | | | |
| Rice *starch* | | | |
| Roman chamomile *flowers* | | | |
| St. John's wort *flowers* | | | |
| Spinach *leaves* | | | |
| Watermelon *fruit* | | | |
| Yarrow *flowers* | | | |

# Cleansing gel with white of egg

*This deep-cleanses the skin of the face, leaving it soft and radiant.*

## INGREDIENTS

1 egg white

¾ tsp/3 g avocado oil

2 tsp/10 g lemon juice

1 oz/25 g refined chickpea flour

10 drops marigold MT

5 drops lemon EO

You should do this very gently, and only if your skin is free of all signs of redness or inflammation.

•

This recipe is only intended as a guide. You can vary it by using chamomile or marigold oil instead of avocado for a more soothing and emollient effect.

•

The mixture will keep for 3–4 days in an airtight container in the refrigerator.

Put the ingredients in a bowl and mix vigorously with a spoon to a very soft, creamy consistency.

•

Spread over the face, massaging gently with the fingertips. Take your time, concentrating on areas with stale make-up or greasy skin.

•

Rinse well with lukewarm water, using a wad of cotton wool/cotton or a sponge, if desired. Repeat if necessary. Dry the face.

•

You can use any size of egg, but the amounts shown are proportional to a small one.

•

Any type of legume flour can be used (bean, pea, lentil, soya bean, lupin, fenugreek, etc.), but it must be refined, not wholemeal.

•

You can use wholemeal flour which, massaged into the skin, will act as an exfoliant – a mild abrasive to peel away the surface skin cells.

# Yogurt cleanser

*Yogurt is one of the few genuinely "live" foods, as it contains* Lactobacillus bulgaricus *and* Streptococcus thermophilus, *whose enzymes are highly beneficial, even when used externally.*

## INGREDIENTS

2 oz/50 g natural yogurt

2 tsp/10 g liquid honey

¾ tsp/3 g wheatgerm oil

1 oz/30 g peeled and very finely sliced apple

1 tsp/4 g lemon juice

⅓ oz/10 g instant-mashed potato or potato flour

15 drops rosemary MT

5 drops lavender EO

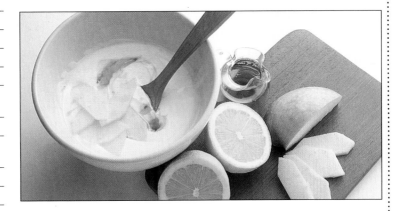

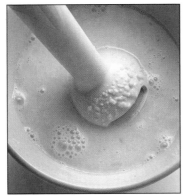

*Put the first five ingredients in a bowl.*

•

*Mix until you reduce the apple to a pulp, using a blender or mashing with a fork.*

•

*Add the potato and mix to a cream with a spoon.*

•

*Add the rosemary and lavender drops and give the mixture a final stir.*

Use the mixture according to the instructions opposite as a cleansing cream. Massage it over the face, paying particular attention to stale make-up, "problem" areas and wrinkles. Use both hands and make gentle but decisive, upward-and-outward, symmetrical movements.

•

Rinse thoroughly with lukewarm water. Repeat if necessary. Dry. People with very dry skin should use jojoba oil instead of wheatgerm.

•

Natural cleansing milks do not usually need to be followed by a toner. However you can make one to suit your skin type.

•

The mixture will keep for 2–3 days in an airtight container in the refrigerator.

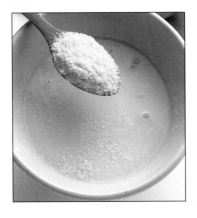

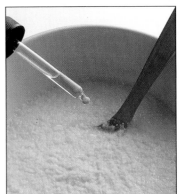

# Honey and vegetable juice

*Honey has been used for cosmetic purposes for thousands of years. If used regularly as a cleanser, it will make the skin soft and velvety.*

### INGREDIENTS

1 oz/30 g pure acacia honey

2 pints/1 liter still mineral water

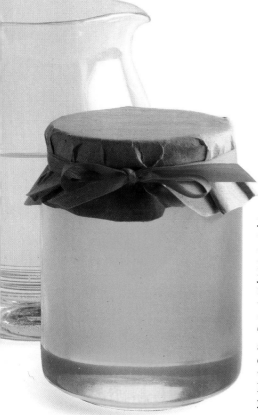

This formula alone is fine especially if you do not have much time, but if you are prepared to spend a little longer on an even better recipe, add 3½ oz/100 g chopped cucumber.

Dissolve the honey in the mineral water. Make sure the water is tepid before using.

If you are adding cucumber, peel, dice and mash 3½ oz/100 g of it with an equivalent volume of mineral water. Alternatively put it in a blender for a minute at low speed and a minute at high speed. Add this pulp to the honey and water mixture.

Use the mixture to give the face a long, thorough wash: it acts as an emollient, clarifier and astringent. You can also prolong the effect by soaking cotton wool/cotton balls or pads in the liquid and placing them on the face.

Add other juices to make your own individual recipe. Potato or carrot juice, for example, alone or in combination, have even better emollient and anti-inflammatory properties. Or the freshly-squeezed juice of one or more citrus fruit makes a good astringent and has a toning effect.

Two tablespoons of cider vinegar are an acceptable substitute and quicker at hand.

For more thorough cleansing, or if you want to use the mixture to wash the body with the aid of a sponge, you can add a tablespoon of rice flour.

The mixture will keep for a maximum of two days, in an airtight container in the refrigerator.

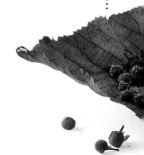

# Cleansing milk with honey

*This is particularly good for cleansing very sensitive skin*
*(once clear of any make-up), including that of infants.*

## INGREDIENTS

| |
|---|
| 2 oz/50 g whole milk (cow's) |
| 1½ oz/40 g pure acacia honey |
| 1 tsp/4 g chamomile oil |
| ⅓ oz/10 g fresh marsh mallow leaves |
| ⅔ oz/20 g refined wheat flour |
| 15 drops chamomile MT |
| 5 drops chamomile or yarrow EO |
| 2 oz/60 g still mineral water |

Simmer the marsh mallow leaves in 2 oz/60 g of water, in a covered pan for 10 minutes. If you use dried leaves, you will need half the amount in 2½ oz/70 g of water. You can use lettuce leaves instead of marsh mallow. Choose the greenest, outer leaves and treat in the same way as fresh marsh mallow.

•

Put all the ingredients in a blender for one minute at high speed. Use the resulting liquid as a normal cleansing milk, massaging with the fingers. Rinse thoroughly with tepid water and repeat if necessary. Concentrate on "problem" areas and dry the face carefully.

•

For a more astringent cleanser, use witch hazel leaves instead of marsh mallow or, for a stronger effect, add 1 oz/30 g of decoction of tormentil roots: use ⅕ oz/5 g of roots and 2½ oz/70 g of water; simmer for 5 minutes in a covered pan.

•

For a creamier mixture, add more flour.

•

It keeps for two days in the refrigerator.

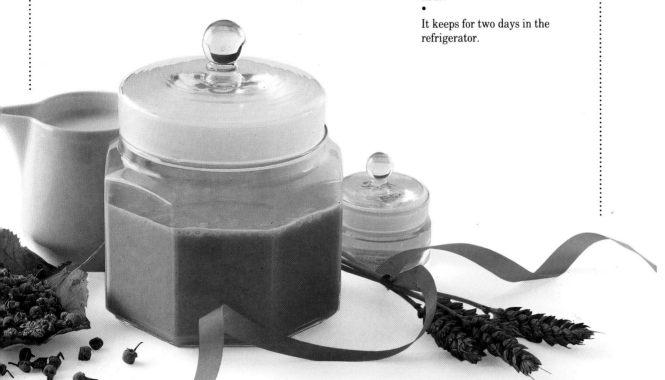

# Anti-wrinkle beauty fluid

*A sixteenth-century herbalist describes this as a "heavenly liquid" with all manner of virtues, which cleansed and softened the skin and made the complexion youthful and radiant.*

## INGREDIENTS

2¾ oz/75 g rye bread without crusts

2 fresh egg whites

1 pint/½ liter cider vinegar

2 oz/50 g tincture of benzoin

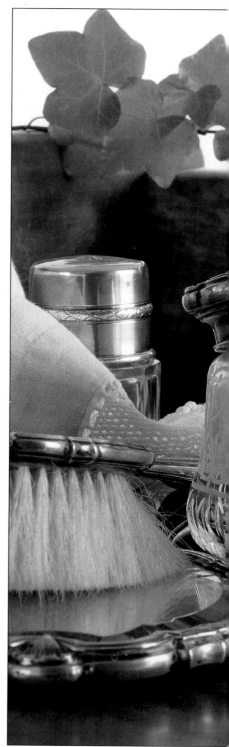

Crumble the bread and soak it overnight in the cider vinegar, in a covered bowl.

•

Pour into a blender, add the egg whites, blend for a minute at low speed and a minute at high speed.

•

Strain through muslin/cheesecloth into a jar, add the tincture of benzoin and shake the mixture thoroughly.

•

This creamy liquid cleans the skin perfectly, lightens it and prevents signs of ageing.

•

You can use it in the bath alone or diluted with water. It will keep for a week in the refrigerator.

•

Tincture of benzoin is an alcoholic mixture based on benzoin, a gum resin secreted by the bark of *Styrax benzoin*. It has a mildly disinfectant and tonic effect on the skin. The best type of benzoin is sold in the form of solidified drops.

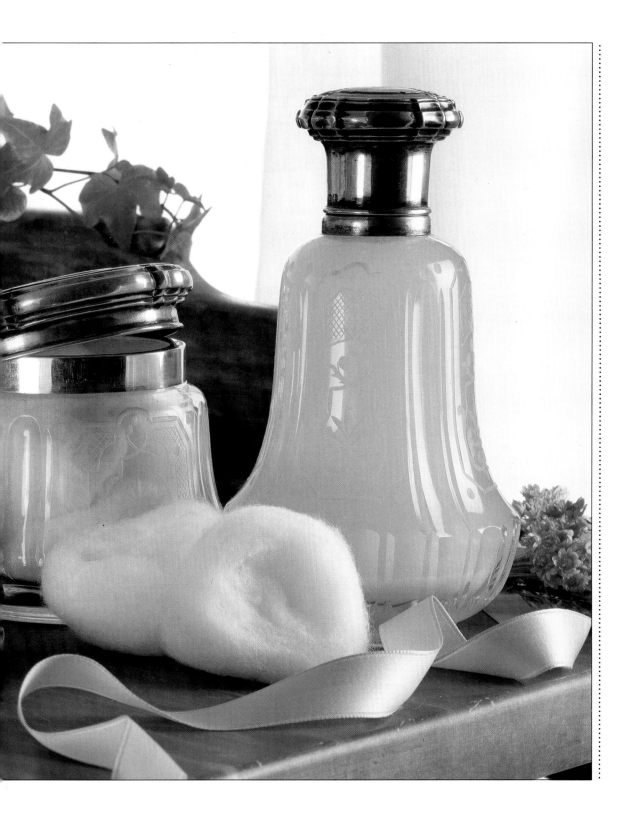

# EXFOLIATION

*Strictly speaking, this describes a process carried out by dermatologists or plastic surgeons. It involves stripping away the top layer of skin, using chemical substances (e.g. resorcinol), abrasive techniques (surgical tools), or physical means (e.g. liquid nitrogen). In the world of cosmetics, exfoliation is a form of deep cleansing which only affects the most superficial layers of the skin. You can use a harmless chemical-enzymatic process, using the juice or flesh of ripe pineapple or unripe papaya. These contain enzymes called bromelain and papain, respectively, which help remove the dead surface cells. You can also use a mildly-abrasive procedure, which consists of massaging unrefined cereal or legume flour or other vegetable or mineral powders very gently into the face.*

*Neither method should be used if you have any spots, sunburn or inflammation of any kind. Do not imagine that you will find a brand new skin underneath: we are not snakes! Follow the directions carefully and use your common sense; after a few tries you will know what is best for your skin. This table lists the main substances that have been used for this purpose in the past. They can be blended to a smooth consistency using a non-proteinaceous binding agent chosen from the list on page 59. Fruit and vegetable flesh or agar-agar, are also suitable.*

---

## PROTEOLYTIC EXFOLIATION
### RIPE PINEAPPLE – UNRIPE PAPAYA

**Parts used**
The juice and flesh

**How?**
Cotton wool/cotton balls or pads soaked in the juice and used as a face pack
The flesh reduced to a pulp and applied to the face

**How long?**
20–30 minutes

---

## ABRASIVE EXFOLIATION

Wholemeal cereal flours
(wheat, millet, oat, barley, rye, maize)

■

Bran

■

Wholemeal legume flours
(chickpea, bean, lentil, pea, soya, fenugreek, lupin)

■

Various types of flour
from seeds (sweet almonds) and roots (iris)

■

Clays

■

Fine cane sugar

■

Diatomaceous earth

■

Extra-fine pumice-stone powder

# Soya facial scrub

*This mildly-abrasive mixture removes the dead cells on the topmost layer of the skin and stimulates the circulation.*

### INGREDIENTS

1 whole egg

½ oz/15 g wholemeal soya flour

2 tsp/10 g extra-virgin olive oil

30 drops marigold MT

30 drops chamomile MT

30 drops witch hazel MT

Mix the ingredients vigorously in a cup, to the consistency of thick cream.

•

Massage gently into the skin with the fingertips, a little at a time, using sinuous, circular movements which follow the lines of the face, from the center outwards. Avoid the lips and area around the eyes.

Rinse with tepid water. Dry and apply a nourishing cream.

•

Several short treatments are better than one long one. Two or three a month are enough, possibly alternated with the recipe overleaf.

•

It will keep for a couple of days in the refrigerator.

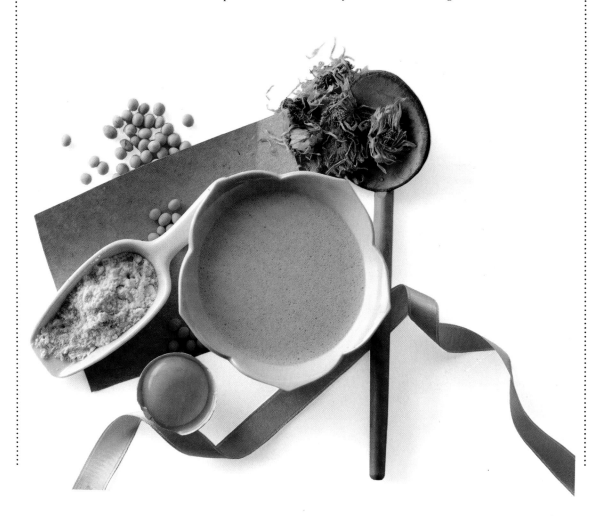

# Pineapple or papaya facial scrub

*This acts by removing a very fine, superficial layer of dead skin cells.*

## INGREDIENTS

3½ oz/100 g ripe pineapple flesh

1½ oz/40 g peeled and cored apple

⅕ oz/5 g white clay

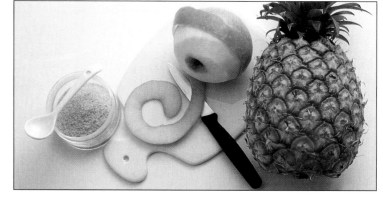

Lie on your back and smooth the cream, made according to the instructions opposite, over the face and neck, or spread it on to pieces of cloth and put them on the face, avoiding the lips and area around the eyes.

•

Relax and leave for 20–30 minutes, then rinse with lukewarm water and dry. Gently massage a nourishing cream into the face.

•

If you prefer not to use the raw fruit, you can soak cotton wool/cotton in pineapple juice instead. Do not forget to avoid the lips and eye area.

•

You can substitute papaya flesh or juice for pineapple. The amounts needed are the same. The effect is stronger if you use unripe fruit.

•

If you do this three times a month, it will greatly improve your complexion. The mixture is active as soon as it is made and should be used immediately, as its properties deteriorate rapidly.

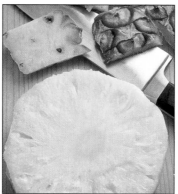

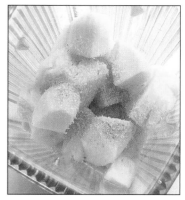

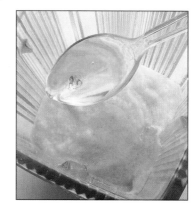

*Peel and core the apple. Cut a thick slice of ripe pineapple and remove the rind.*

•

*Dice both and put in a blender with the white clay.*

•

*Blend for a minute at low speed and a minute at high speed.*

•

*If the mixture is too thick, add a teaspoonful of liquid honey.*

## FACE MASKS

*The face mask is one of the oldest, simplest and most effective beauty treatments. The following ones use the edible ingredients listed under cleansing milks on page 61. The only difference is that you need thicker, creamier mixtures, which are spread over a clean face, left to act for 20–30 minutes, then rinsed off. Nearly all animal and vegetable fats have cleansing, emollient and nourishing properties, as do many oily fruits, like avocado pears and almonds. The starch in flour, cellulose gels and starchy fruit and vegetables (like bananas and potatoes) are cleansing, emollient and soothing, and thus good for many types of skin irritation. The flesh and juice of moist fruit and vegetables have been used for cosmetic purposes for thousands of years, as they are full of vitamins, mineral salts, organic acids and other useful substances. Some are emollient and soften the skin, while others are astringent. Some stimulate the circulation, while others whiten the skin or act as disinfectants. With practice, you will learn how to use this range of properties harmoniously. One last word of advice: relaxation is a vital part of any beauty treatment. Treat the time spent making your own cosmetics as an opportunity to unwind. Face masks are ideal for this, as you generally need to lie down while they take effect.*

# Marsh mallow face mask

*Marsh mallow leaves are very good for sensitive skin. You can use either fresh or dried ones.*

## INGREDIENTS

4 tsp/20 g untreated acacia honey

2 tsp/10 g almond oil

⅔ oz/20 g fresh marsh mallow leaves

⅓ oz/10 g wheat starch

20 drops blackcurrant MG

5 drops peppermint EO

4½ oz/30 g still mineral water

Simmer the marsh mallow leaves gently in a covered pan for 10 minutes until nearly all the water has gone.
If using dried leaves, use ⅓ oz/10 g with 5 oz/150 g water.

•

Blend all the ingredients in a blender for one minute.

•

Smooth over the face and neck, or any area which has been irritated by the sun, wind or other factors.

•

Leave for at least half an hour, then rinse with tepid water and dry.

•

It makes the skin beautifully soft and relieves inflammation in young and old alike.
It keeps for a day or two in the refrigerator.

•

Tender young marsh mallow leaves can be added to salads, soups or sautéed with vegetables like spinach.

# Apple face mask

*Countless recipes for cosmetics have been based on apples.*
*Some have survived from the remote past. The word*
*"pomade" originally meant a preparation containing apples.*

## INGREDIENTS

| |
|---|
| 5 oz/150 g apple flesh |
| 4 tsp/20 g lemon juice |
| 2 tsp/10 g almond oil |
| 2 tsp/10 g wheatgerm oil |
| ⅓ oz/10 g egg white |
| 20 drops marigold EO |

Peel and core a ripe apple. Remove any discoloured parts. Dice and place in the blender with the other ingredients.

•

Blend for a minute at low speed and a minute at high speed.

•

Spread the resulting cream ⅛ in (2–3 mm) thick over the face and neck (having removed all traces of make-up).

•

Depending on the amount of juice in the apple, the cream may be too wet or too dry. If so, add a teaspoon of rice flour or more lemon juice, as appropriate, blending for another minute.

•

Lie back and relax for at least half an hour, then rinse off with tepid water and dry.

•

Apples are very good for you, whether eaten or used externally, as the pulp contains mucilage, pectin, organic acids, vitamins and mineral salts. So use one for the face mask, and eat one. It will help improve the complexion and counteract the damage inflicted on your skin by the weather and the vicissitudes of life.

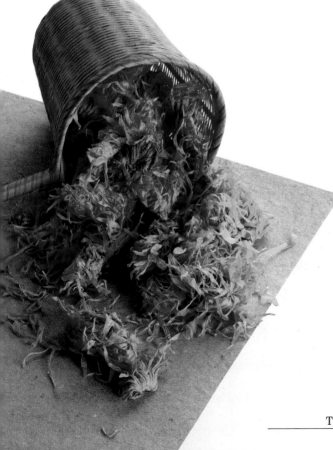

# Face cream with buds and beeswax

*You can use this recipe as the basis for a number of face creams, using different types of bud for different skin problems.*

## INGREDIENTS

⅓ oz/10 g pure beeswax

½ oz/15 g cocoa butter

1 oz/30 g sweet almond oil

4 tsp/20 g avocado oil

⅔ oz/20 g lime/linden or poplar bud MG

2 tsp/10 g acacia honey

50 drops rose EO

Using a double boiler or a stainless steel saucepan and bowl, dissolve the beeswax and cocoa butter in the oils.

•

Add the macerated glycerine and honey.

•

Remove from heat. Replace the boiling water in the double boiler with cold.

•

Blend with an electric beater. The mixture should turn creamy as it cools.

•

Add the essential oil of roses (or another perfume, if preferred) and blend carefully.

•

Put into clean, 1-fl oz/30-ml airtight bottles and refrigerate.

•

Lime/linden buds increase the emollient and healing properties of the cream. Blackcurrant buds help guard against allergies, while horse-chestnut and black poplar are good for blotchy skin.

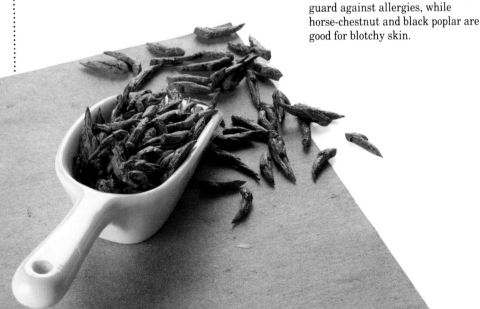

# Steam treatment with herbs and a face mask

*This deep-cleans the skin and is good for acne and greasy skin, as it frees the sebaceous ducts and hair follicles of impurities. It is disinfectant and astringent.*

## INGREDIENTS

| |
|---|
| ⅔ oz/20 g marigold flowers |
| ⅓ oz/10 g chamomile flowers |
| ⅓ oz/10 g lavender flowers |
| ⅓ oz/10 g marjoram leaves |
| ⅓ oz/10 g walnut leaves |
| ⅓ oz/10 g rosemary leaves |
| ⅓ oz/10 g sage leaves |
| ⅓ oz/10 g lime/linden flowers |
| ⅓ oz/10 g thyme leaves |
| 4 pints/2 liters mineral water for the face mask |
| ⅔ oz/20 g clay |
| 30 drops witch hazel MT |

Follow the directions opposite. Keeping at a safe distance so as not to scald yourself, let the steam act for as long as it lasts. Then rinse your face with hot water and dry it.

•

Mix the clay with two tablespoons of the infusion, to a thick but not stiff, cream.

•

Spread over the face ⅛ in (1–2 mm) thick, and leave for at least half an hour. Use your fingers or a brush.

•

If you have acne or very greasy skin, leave the clay on until it dries and "pulls" the skin. This way it will absorb more oil. Otherwise, keep it moist by putting paper tissue or cotton wool/cotton pads soaked in the infusion on top.

•

By repeating this mask often (up to three times a week), you can avoid ever needing to squeeze pores, which can often rupture delicate capillaries.

•

Rinse away all traces of the mixture with lukewarm water and dry the face.

•

Use a cooling toner like cucumber juice, or grape or tomato juice on a piece of cotton wool/cotton, to which a few drops of oil have been added, for example, 2 drops of almond oil and 3 of jojoba (dry skin), or 3 drops of avocado oil and 2 of evening primrose (ageing skin), to each piece of soaked cotton wool/cotton.

Pat over the face gently working it in with the fingertips. Pat dry with a tissue.

•

Always dry the skin carefully. You should never leave any liquid (water, tonic or other) to dry by evaporation.

•

Finish by gently applying a nourishing cream (for normal, dry or oily skin) or use a propolis pomade (for acne).

•

Steam treatments are not recommended for people with blotchy skin or broken veins.

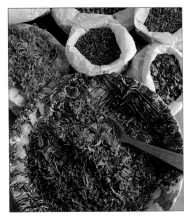

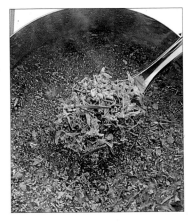

*Measure the herbs carefully and combine in a bowl. Boil the water and add three heaped tablespoons of the herbs. Remove from heat immediately and cover.*

*Wait for 10 minutes, then place the pan on a table where you can safely and comfortably sit over it.*

*Remove the saucepan lid and lean over the steam, putting a large towel over the head and saucepan to stop the steam escaping.*

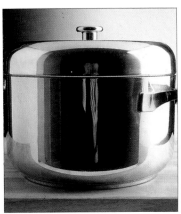

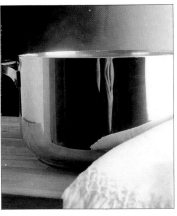

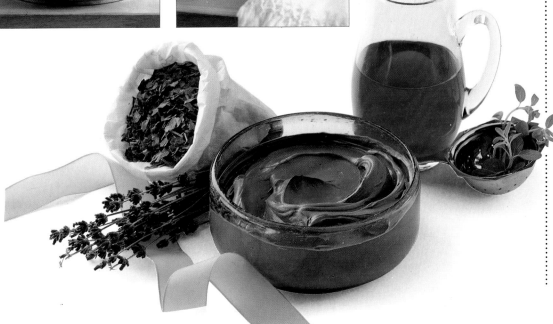

# Live yogurt and yeast mask

*This is suitable for all types of skin and is full of enzymes which are good for the complexion.*

## INGREDIENTS

1 oz/30 g whole milk natural yogurt

4 tsp/20 g pure acacia honey

2 tsp/10 g sweet almond oil

⅔ oz/20 g melon flesh

⅕ oz/5 g marsh mallow leaves (dried)

½ oz/15 g kaolin

⅔ oz/30 g brewer's yeast

3¼ oz/90 g still mineral water

Simmer the marsh mallow leaves in a stainless steel pan for about 10 minutes, until they absorb all the water.

•

Put them in a blender with the other ingredients and run it for a minute at low speed and a minute at high speed.

•

If you use fresh marsh mallow leaves, you will need ⅓ oz/10 g and only ¾ of the water. You can use green lettuce or beet leaves as an alternative, and marrow/squash or cucumber flesh instead of melon.

•

The mixture should have the consistency of thick cream. Add extra yeast and kaolin if needed.

Lie back and spread the mixture over the face. Or you can cut a "face mask" out of a piece of cotton fabric or cheese cloth, with holes for eyes, nose and mouth. Spread the mixture on this and lay it on the face. Leave on for half an hour.

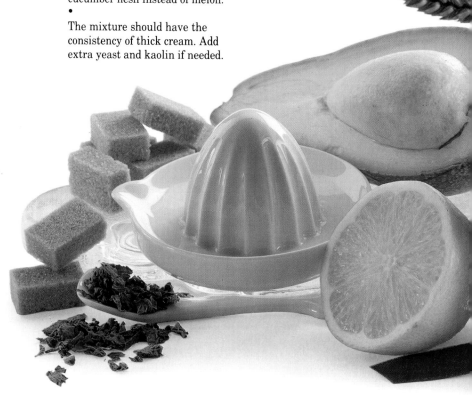

# Nourishing face mask with avocado

*This fruit makes a very nourishing and regulating face mask
on its own. The other ingredients enhance its properties.*

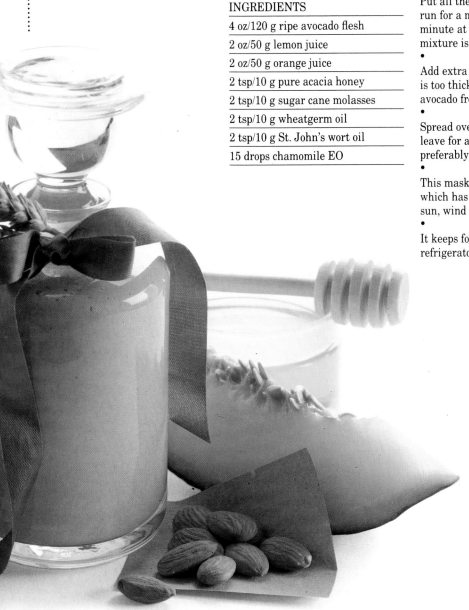

### INGREDIENTS

| |
|---|
| 4 oz/120 g ripe avocado flesh |
| 2 oz/50 g lemon juice |
| 2 oz/50 g orange juice |
| 2 tsp/10 g pure acacia honey |
| 2 tsp/10 g sugar cane molasses |
| 2 tsp/10 g wheatgerm oil |
| 2 tsp/10 g St. John's wort oil |
| 15 drops chamomile EO |

Put all the ingredients in a blender, run for a minute at low speed and a minute at high speed, until the mixture is smooth and creamy.

•

Add extra orange or lemon juice if it is too thick. These also prevent the avocado from turning black.

•

Spread over the face and neck and leave for at least 30 minutes, preferably longer.

•

This mask is excellent for skin which has been exposed to too much sun, wind or cold weather.

•

It keeps for a day or two in the refrigerator.

# Fruit face mask

*This is nourishing, firming, soothing and healing, even for dull and lifeless, or blotchy and irritated skin.*

## INGREDIENTS

1 oz/25 g whole milk natural yogurt

4 tsp/20 g pure acacia honey

4 tsp/20 g apple flesh

4 tsp/20 g banana flesh

4 tsp/20 g plum flesh

6 tsp/30 g apricot flesh

⅓ oz/10 g orris root powder

4 tsp/20 g yarrow oil

30 drops lime/linden bud MG

Peel the fruit, remove seeds and any discoloured parts; chop and place in a blender with the other ingredients. Blend for a minute at low speed and a minute at high speed.

•

If the fruit was very juicy and the mixture is too runny, add extra orris root powder. This should be very fine. If not, sieve it, shaking the sieve from side to side.

•

This mixture should be used fresh, as it only keeps for a day.

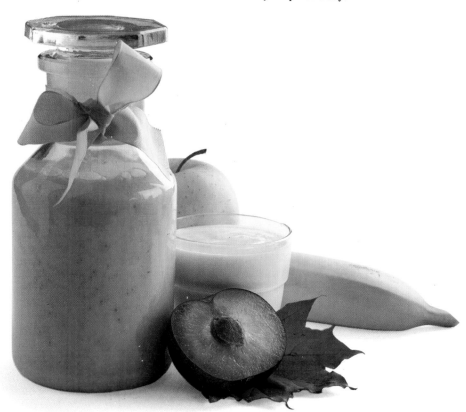

Cosmetic waters can be made at home and used on their own or as ingredients for other cosmetics (e.g. face masks, lotions). The recipes explain how to extract the active principles from herbs, always using still mineral water as a solvent. The rose and orange flower waters that you can buy in stores are produced in special distilling apparatus. Plant parts are exposed to a draught of aqueous steam, at a temperature of 212°F/100°C, which causes them to release their perfume. When the steam condenses, small quantities of essential oil are obtained, together with a lot of distilled water, in which traces, or minute amounts, of essential oil are dissolved.

The cosmetic waters described here are produced by infusion, decoction, maceration or squeezing. They should be patted on to a clean face with the fingers, or applied with cotton wool/cotton or in a fine spray. Skin should always be carefully dried afterwards. The skin absorbs the active principles of the plants used to make them, and they act as the finishing touch to your face cleansing, softening and clarifying it. The table on page 59 lists a number of plants and fruits in groups according to their cosmetic uses. This gives a good idea of the properties to be found in the various ingredients of the following recipes.

# Emollient skin toner

*This completes the process of cleansing the face and makes the skin soft and velvety.*

## INGREDIENTS

⅓ oz/10 g lime/linden flowers with bracts (the small leaves often found at the base of flower stalks)

⅓ oz/10 g marsh mallow flowers

⅓ oz/10 g elder flowers

3 pints/1¾ liter still mineral water

Boil the ingredients in a stainless steel pan and simmer for 5 minutes.
•
Remove from the heat and cover. Strain through a fine sieve when tepid.
•
Use as skin toner, facial cleanser in the morning, or as a refreshing face pack. In the latter case, soak sterile cotton wool/cotton pads in the mixture and lay it on the face, neck and eyelids. Leave to act for 5 to 15 minutes.
•
It only keeps for a day or two in the refrigerator.
•
Always dry the skin carefully after using a toner.
•
Marsh mallow and elder can also be used in cooking. Delicious jams, cordials and wine are made from elder berries. Marsh mallow leaves can be eaten in salads and soups.

# Vegetable toner

*Freshly-squeezed vegetable juice, like fruit juice, is a "live" food, packed with health-giving substances: it will not take long before you begin to feel the benefits.*

## INGREDIENTS

2 oz/50 g cucumber flesh

2 oz/50 g green lettuce leaves

2 oz/50 g lemon juice

2 oz/50 g tomato flesh

You can make your own vegetable toner by extracting juices in a juice extractor or mixing chopped raw vegetables in a blender and straining the pulp.
•

Although these vegetable juices mainly consist of water, they are quite different from tapwater. Theirs is a biological fluid, composed of cellular juices and lymph, a type of vegetable blood full of living substances which are highly beneficial, even when used externally.
•

They will keep for a couple of days in the refrigerator, but are best used immediately.
•

The cucumber is an emollient as well as a tonic. You can make face masks and pomades with the juice. It is widely used in cosmetics to lighten the colour of the skin.
•

The tomato contains vitamin A, riboflavin and vitamin C and is thus ideal for cosmetic as well as culinary purposes.

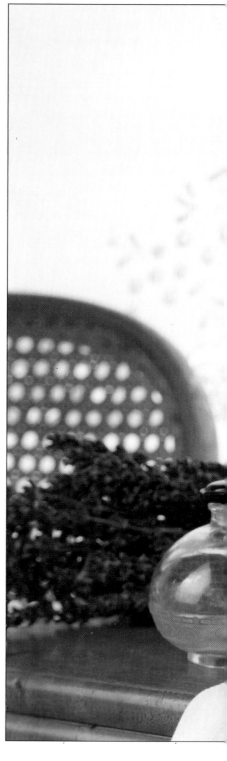

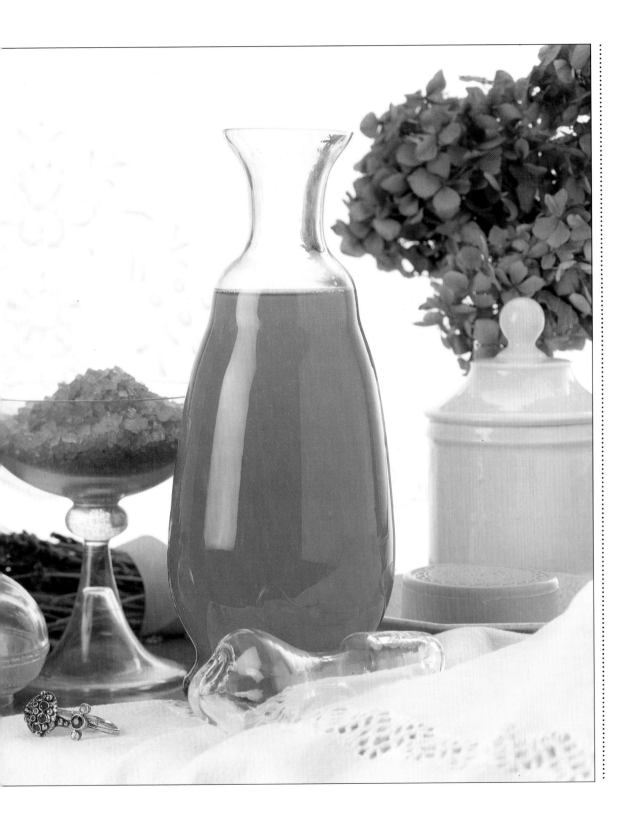

# Rosemary toner

*According to a sixteenth-century herbalist, rosemary flowers boiled in white wine make a good tonic for the complexion and also an excellent drink which sweetens the breath.*

## INGREDIENTS

1 oz/30 g rosemary flowers

2 pints/1 liter dry white wine

Put the wine and flowers in a stainless steel pan and gently bring to the boil.
•

Simmer for three minutes with the lid half on, then remove from heat and cover, until tepid, before straining.
•

Use alone as an occasional, mildly-alcoholic toner. It is also good to tone the scalp and the whole body. A tablespoonful in a glass of water makes a good gargle.
•

It has antiseptic, healing, stimulating and anti-wrinkle properties. It will keep in a cool, dark place, if stored in small, airtight bottles.
•

For a stronger tonic best used for oily hair and scalp add extracts of nettle and cinchona, or add EO of marjoram, thyme, sage or eucalyptus, which have stronger antiseptic and deodorant properties.

You can also boil other flowers in the wine (same quantities, same time), for example: elder and rose flowers (astringent and clarifying); orange and lime flowers (toning); chamomile (softening and soothing); hop (firming).
•

If the toner should turn vinegary, you can always use it as an after-shampoo rinse or a mouthwash.

# Fruit toner

*Succulent fruit juices make perfect skin toners, used alone or in combinations. This has long been appreciated for there are few other foods at table which you can eat and drink while at the same time washing your face!*

### INGREDIENTS

| |
|---|
| 2 oz/50 g orange juice |
| 2 oz/50 g strawberry flesh |
| 2 oz/50 g apple flesh |
| 2 oz/50 g cherry flesh |

Put all the ingredients in a blender and run it for a minute at low speed and a minute at high speed.

•

Pour the resultant creamy liquid into a muslin or cheesecloth bag the size of a trouser pocket. It should pass through quickly. Squeeze the bag for excess liquid.

•

If you double the recipe, drink a glassful, for the vitamins, mineral salts and other beneficial substances. Used externally it makes a very good tonic which, if used regularly, can make the skin soft and radiant.

•

It is best if used immediately, although it will keep for a day.

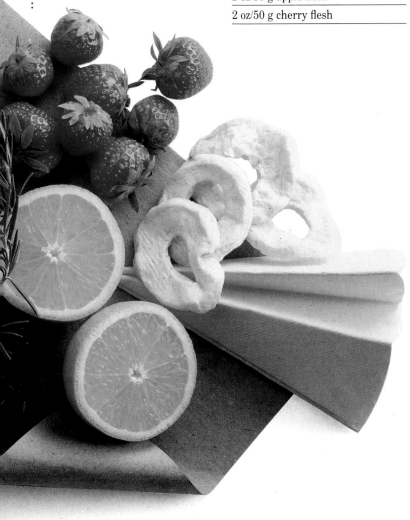

# Oily skin toner

*The plants used for this act as a tonic and an astringent and help control excess oiliness.*

### INGREDIENTS

| |
|---|
| 1 oz/30 g horsetail (stalks) |
| $2/3$ oz/20 g Iceland moss |
| $2/3$ oz/20 g witch hazel (leaves) |
| 3 pints/1¾ liter still mineral water |

Boil the ingredients in a stainless steel pan and simmer for 5 minutes. Remove from heat and cover.
•
Leave to soak overnight.
•
The following morning, simmer the mixture for another 5 minutes, remove from heat and leave covered until tepid. Strain through a fine sieve.
•
This is a good emollient, astringent and corrective toner for oily skin, even skin with acne. It can also be used as a face pack to firm and tone flaccid skin, possibly with the addition of female hop inflorescence and extract of ginseng.
•
It keeps for a day or two refrigerated in sealed glass bottles.
•
A decoction of Iceland moss in a drink is very good for persistent coughs. Add a teaspoon per cup of water or milk, simmer for five minutes and sweeten with honey.
•
Horsetail is also used in homeopathy to treat urine infections by increasing urination.

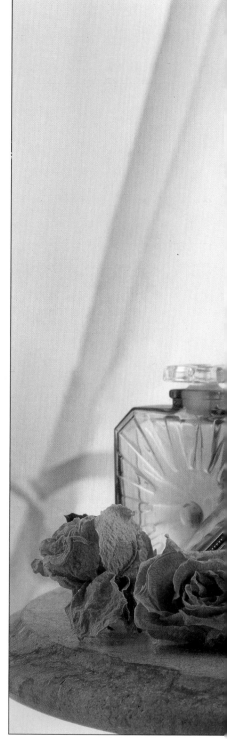

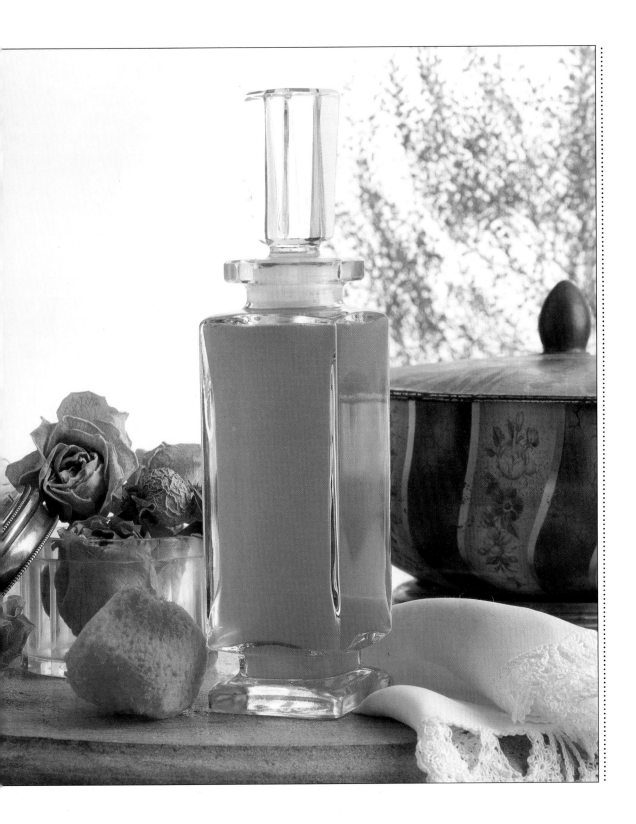

Creams and pomades are very easy to make, but much harder to keep, without using anti-bacterial and anti-fungal agents and all the other substances which are added to the mass-produced varieties to preserve them.

Many essential oils act as good disinfectants, but they must be used sparingly, as they can be overpowering. Also, at high doses they can cause allergic reactions and some are photosensitive. It is best, therefore, to make just a little of these recipes at a time according to your needs.

Anhydrous creams, or those that do not contain water, can be stored in the butter compartment of the fridge. The jar in immediate use can be kept at room temperature. If you make a large batch, you can freeze some of the pots.

Store creams least likely to keep in small (1-fl oz/30-ml) jars. The creams in the following recipes are nourishing; if used in small amounts and smoothed in carefully, they have the same effect as moisturizing creams. Even people with oily skin will benefit from using them on a regular basis, unlike the moisturizers you can buy which tend to aggravate the condition known as reactive seborrhea (over-stimulated oil glands).

As with all the recipes in this book, you can learn the basic techniques from these pages and then, with experience, vary them to suit your personal requirements.

# Moisturizing cream

*This cream was first made by Galen, the Greek physician, in the third century. The Americans renamed it "cold cream," and it is still widely used today.*

## INGREDIENTS

| ½–⅔ oz/18 g beeswax |
| 2¼ oz/60 g sweet almond oil |
| 4 tsp/20 g rosewater |
| ½ tsp/2 g soya lecithin |
| 5 drops rose EO |

Put the first four ingredients in a small enamel, stainless steel or glass container and melt the wax and lecithin by standing it in a saucepan of hot water.

•

When completely liquid, mix vigorously with a spoon or electric beater.

•

Replace the hot water in the saucepan with cold, and continue mixing until the mixture is cooler and starts to thicken.

•

The water underneath will have absorbed heat from the mixture, so replace it again with cold water. Add the essential oil of roses to the cream and mix again.

•

When the cream has reached the right consistency, put it into clean, airtight jars and refrigerate.

•

This does not keep as long as the nourishing cream opposite, as this one contains water. Therefore use spotlessly clean implements and containers to avoid the fungus spores and bacteria of dust and dirt which deteriorate the cream. Make small amounts and refrigerate.

# Nourishing cream

*This is suitable for all complexions, including oily skin, as it has an emollient, protective and balancing effect.*

### INGREDIENTS

⅓ oz/10 g cocoa butter

⅓ oz/10 g pure beeswax

½ tsp/2 g soya lecithin

1 oz/30 g sweet almond oil

2 tsp/10 g avocado oil

2 tsp/10 g wheatgerm oil

2 tsp/10 g thick honey

⅓ oz/10 g lime/linden bud MG

5 drops lemon EO

3 drops lemon verbena EO

Put the first six ingredients in a double boiler or stainless steel pan over another pan of boiling water.
•

Dissolve, then stir until well mixed. (You can use an electric beater for this.) Add the honey and lime/linden, still stirring vigorously. Remove from the heat and replace the boiling water in the outer container with cold.
•

Stand the inner container in what is now a cooling bath, stirring constantly. The oily liquid will gradually turn into an opaque cream. When this happens, add one or more essential oils, to perfume it. (Take care to keep to the quantities specified as some essential oils can be photosensitive and cause permanent discoloration of the skin if you sunbathe or use a sun lamp.)

Change the water again, to keep it cold. Continue mixing, until the cream is lukewarm.
•

Put it into new, airtight jars, using a knife or small spatula. Refrigerate to set.
•

The jar in use can safely be kept at room temperature unless your house is very hot.
•

Do not dip into the jar with your fingers. Use the tip of a knife or teaspoon, as this is less likely to introduce bacteria.
•

Massage small amounts gently into clean skin.

# Emollient cream

*This is very good for dry and sensitive skin, including that of infants. It protects the face against the elements.*

### INGREDIENTS

½ oz/15 g pure beeswax

⅓ oz/10 g cocoa butter

¼ tsp/1 g soya lecithin

2 tsp/10 g jojoba oil

2 tsp/10 g avocado oil

2 tsp/10 g marigold oil

½ tsp/1 g white clay

⅕ oz/5 g horsetail stems

⅕ oz/5 g still mineral water

1 drop clove EO

4 drops orange EO

Follow the instructions opposite precisely. Replace the water in a bain-marie or double boiler with fresh, cold water and give the cream a final mix with the electric beater. Keep refrigerated in clean, airtight jars.

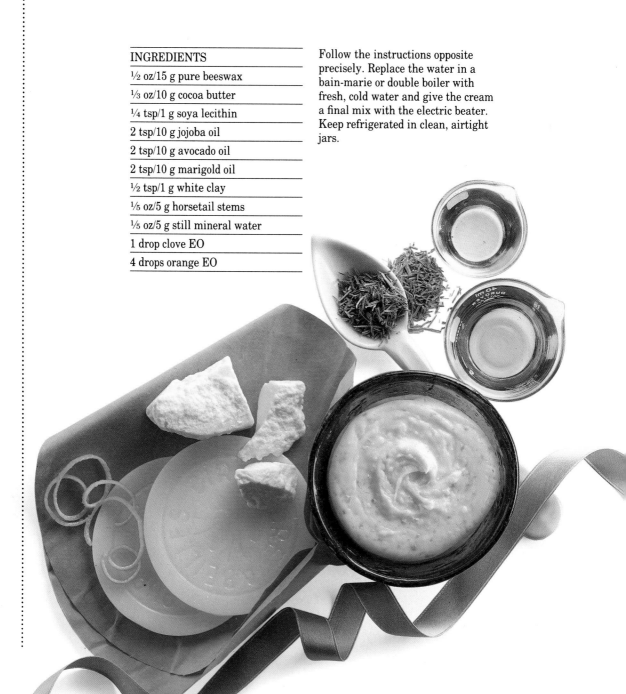

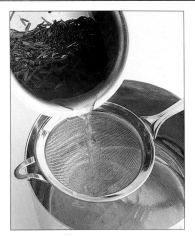

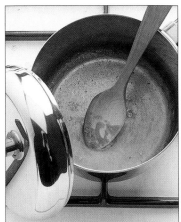

*Put the water and horsetail in a stainless steel pan, bring to a boil and simmer for five minutes. Remove from heat and let stand covered until lukewarm.*

•

*Strain the decoction into another saucepan, add the white clay and blend.*

•

*Stirring constantly, bring the resulting gel gently to a boil and simmer for three minutes. Remove from the heat and let stand covered until lukewarm.*

•

*Put the first seven ingredients in another pan and dissolve by the bain-marie method.*

•

*Add the decoction to these ingredients. Mix with an electric beater. Remove from the heat, replace the boiling water in the outer container with cold. Continue blending until the mixture thickens as it cools. Add the essential oils.*

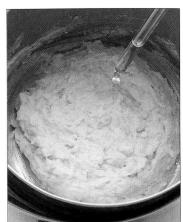

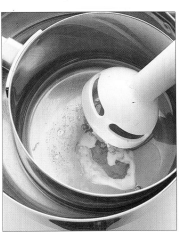

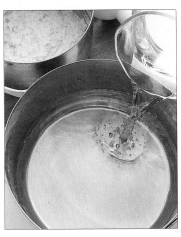

# COSMETICS FOR THE EYES AND MOUTH

*Our most highly-developed sense is that of sight. Never has it been so much abused as in the last century. We have replaced the natural, 24-hour rhythm, marked by the sun's rising and setting, with arbitrary periods of artificial light. In so doing, we have reduced our hours of rest. Many of us work in environments which do nothing to help preserve the eyesight. Offices are illuminated by diffuse, fluorescent lighting, which is not good for reading. Many of us spend a lot of time focusing on things at the same distance.*

*The computer screen is no better for us. Dust, smoke and fumes irritate the eyes still further, both at work and in polluted towns and cities. These concrete jungles lack the restful greens of the woods and fields, green being the colour to which we are genetically predisposed.*

*Our choice of leisure activities does not help either. Most of us spend hours in front of the television or in places with artificial lighting. We take our holidays on sun-drenched beaches or snow-covered mountains, even though one ethologist described people as "apes of the shade" because their natural habitat was the woods and forest margins.*

*We are not taught how to relax when using our eyes. There are simple exercises one can do which would in many cases delay or prevent the downward spiral of dependency on eye glasses. Furthermore, we do not eat enough raw fruit and vegetables, which contain vitamins needed for good eyesight. Instead, we apply eye make-up which can irritate the eyes and cause allergies. It is hardly surprising that opticians are doing a booming trade.*

*In terms of cosmetics, remember that the eyes are vulnerable, and you should only use the very mildest ingredients, like the ones suggested here, on the delicate area of skin around the eyes.*

## The mouth

*The mouth has benefited from improved standards of health and hygiene, but has suffered from changes in our eating habits. From early childhood, many of us have grown accustomed to all kinds of sugary food and drinks, to the point of addiction. These "junk foods" have replaced the fruit, bread and dairy produce which used to be eaten at meal and snack times.*

*Spend 4–5 minutes brushing your teeth systematically. Be sure to use a toothbrush that is in perfect condition and a very small amount of toothpaste. Learn how to use dental floss properly as well. Soft toothpicks and a dental spray will remove particles of food which, if left in the mouth at body temperature would harbour bacteria and form "plaque," the thin film which coats the teeth.*

*The lips are the part of our body which ages the least, possibly because they are always in movement; our lips are able to modulate sounds with such precision that the deaf can "read" what we are saying, just by watching them.*

*Today's lip cosmetics are healthier than ever. People used to underestimate the toxicity of certain dyes, like cinnabar red, an ore of mercury which is poisonous. The sensitive mucous membranes of the lips react to unfamiliar substances like food additives, medicines, cosmetics and pollution. Extremes of climate are also bad for them. They "protest" by swelling and cracking. The lipsticks suggested here are emollient and protective and, because they are edible, are not likely to irritate or cause allergic reactions. If you have very sensitive lips, you can leave out the essential oils. If the idea of colouring them appeals to you, be sure to use only edible colorants.*

# Pomade for the eye area

*Used regularly, this softens wrinkles, crow's feet and other flaws.*

### INGREDIENTS

| |
|---|
| 2 tsp/10 g avocado oil |
| 2 tsp/10 g marigold oil |
| 2 tsp/10 g carrot oil |
| 2 tsp/10 g cod liver oil |
| 2 tsp/10 g wheatgerm oil |
| 2 tsp/10 g St. John's wort oil |
| 2 tsp/10 g castor oil |
| ⅓ oz/10 g beeswax |
| ⅔ oz/10 g cocoa butter |
| 1 tsp/5 g liquid honey |

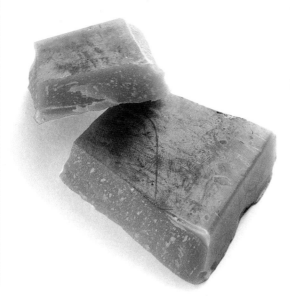

Put the ingredients in a double boiler, or a stainless steel pan in a pan of water, and melt the beeswax and cocoa butter over a low heat.
•

Replace the boiling water in the bain-marie outer pan, with cold and mix the oily liquid in the top pan with a spoon or whisk, until creamy.
•

Replace the cooling bath again, stir the mixture thoroughly and pour it into small, airtight jars, which should be refrigerated. The one in use can be kept at room temperature.
•

The density of the ingredients can vary. If the cream is too runny, you can remelt it and add another ⅓ oz/10 g cocoa butter.
•

The cream has a golden colour; if this does not suit your skin type, leave out the carrot and St. John's wort oils and substitute similar quantities of sweet almond and jojoba oil. If the cod liver oil smells fishy, halve the dose.
Gently smooth a little of the cream around the eye area at night, using the tip of one finger.

# Compress for tired eyes

*This is good for eye strain caused by too much reading or exposure to the sun or wind.*

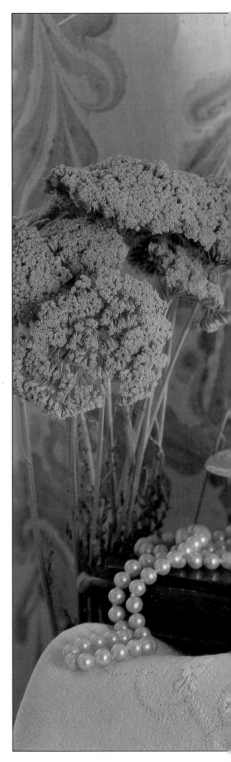

### INGREDIENTS

⅓ oz/10 g marigold flowers

⅕ oz/5 g lavender flowers

⅓ oz/10 g marsh mallow leaves

⅕ oz/5 g walnut leaves

7 oz/200 g still mineral water

Other mixtures of herbs can be used, for example: ⅓ oz/10 g each of kidney vetch flowering heads, marigold flowers, chamomile flowers, fennel seeds and marsh mallow flowers; or ⅓ oz/10 g each of cornflower flowers, licorice root infusion and marsh mallow leaves, with ⅕ oz/5 g black tea. Add a teaspoon of either of these mixtures to boiling water. Simmer for 3 minutes, remove from the heat and cover. Strain after 10 minutes.

Mix the quantities of herbs together and store in a dry place, in sealed paper bags.
To use, bring the water to the boil in a stainless steel pan and add a teaspoon of the mixed herbs. Remove from the heat immediately and cover. Strain into a cup after 10 minutes and use the infusion for compresses during the day.
•
Rather than making fresh amounts every time, you can freeze some of the mixture in ice cube trays. If you melt a couple of cubes a day, it can last all week.
•
Use sterile cotton wool/cotton pads for the compresses. To sterilize cotton wool/cotton balls, boil gently, in a covered stainless steel pan for 15 minutes. Use mineral water. (Tapwater is not suitable because it is usually too hard and may be chlorinated.) Let stand until lukewarm, then remove two cotton wool/cotton balls – one for each eye – with a fork. The rest will remain sterile until you use them.

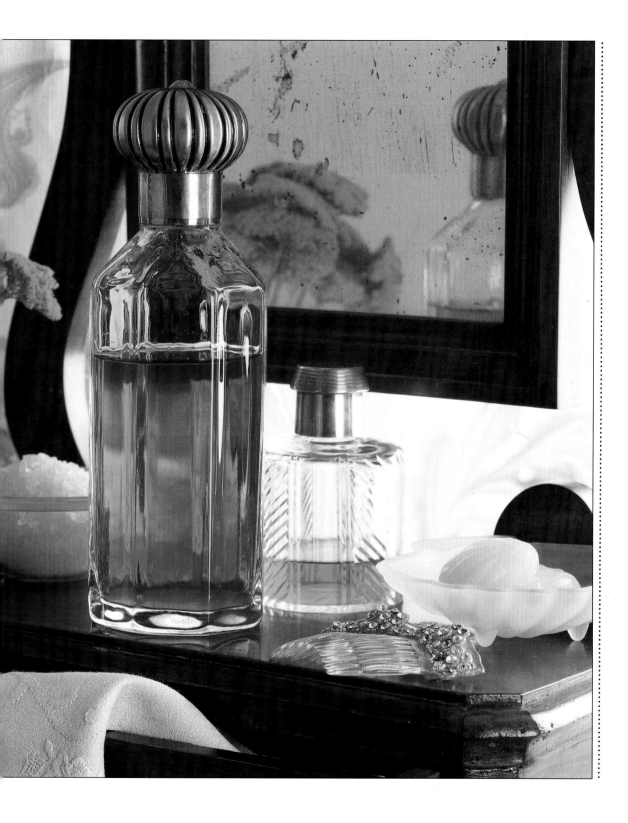

# Lip salve

*The lips can get very dry in the sun, wind or an arid climate.*
*This special lipstick will protect them.*

## INGREDIENTS

½ oz/15 g cocoa butter

⅔ oz/20 g beeswax

2 tsp/10 g avocado oil

2 tsp/10 g wheatgerm oil

2 tsp/10 g castor oil

5 drops rose EO

3 drops chamomile EO

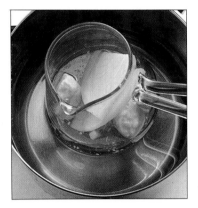

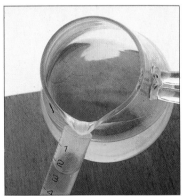

After a few attempts and some experience at measuring, you will become skilled at making numerous lip salves with the recipe described below.

*Put all the ingredients except the essential oils into a small pan with a spout (or use a stainless steel ladle with a lip). Melt over a pan of water.*

*As soon as they have dissolved to an oily liquid, remove from the heat, add the essential oils and stir carefully.*

*Pour into moulds.*
*You can use any cylindrical-shaped mould or small, sealable dishes. Make sure your container is spotlessly clean.*

*Leave the mixture to set for 5 minutes in the freezer or 10 minutes in the refrigerator.*
*A cylindrical-shaped lip salve can be*

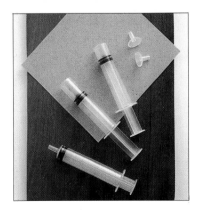

*stored in an old lipstick holder. Store the ones not in use in the refrigerator.*

*As the balm contains no water, the jar you are using may be kept at room temperature.*

# Sage tooth powder

*Tooth powders were used long before the invention of the toothbrush; they were rubbed over the teeth with one finger.*

## INGREDIENTS

⅔ oz/20 g airfloat clay

⅓ oz/10 g powdered orris root

⅔ oz/20 g marsh mallow leaves

1 oz/30 g sage leaves

⅔ oz/20 g lime/linden flowers

20 drops peppermint or aniseed EO
(use aniseed essential oil if you
are taking homeopathic remedies)

Blend the dried herbs in a blender for a minute at low speed and a minute at high speed.
•
The resulting powder should be passed through a very fine sieve several times, a little at a time. Put the powder into a plastic bottle, add the airfloat clay, which is like face powder, and the oil of peppermint or aniseed. Mix by shaking the bottle. Use it as a normal toothpaste, brushing twice: put half a teaspoon of powder in the palm of the hand; use half on a damp toothbrush to clean the teeth; rinse your mouth and then repeat with the other half; rinse several times, brushing between each rinse.
•
Still use dental floss for a more thorough clean, or as directed by your dentist, and finish up with a mouthwash.

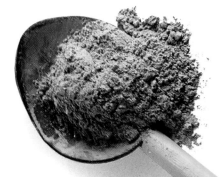

# Propolis stick

*Propolis is a powerful anti-inflammatory agent. It is very good at healing cracks and minor skin irritations and is an effective treatment for cold sores.*

## INGREDIENTS

1 tsp/4 g sweet almond oil

1 tsp/4 g olive oil

1 tsp/4 g wheatgerm oil

⅓ oz/10 g cocoa butter

⅓ oz/10 g beeswax

⅕ oz/5 g raw propolis

Melt the ingredients in a double boiler or small stainless steel pan in a pan of water.

Stir constantly with a spatula. Only a little of the propolis will blend with the other ingredients; most of it will turn creamy but stay at the bottom of the pan.

Pour the liquid into moulds (see recipe on p. 94) and refrigerate. The propolis on the bottom of the pan can be reused.

You can make these into coloured lip balms by adding food colour.

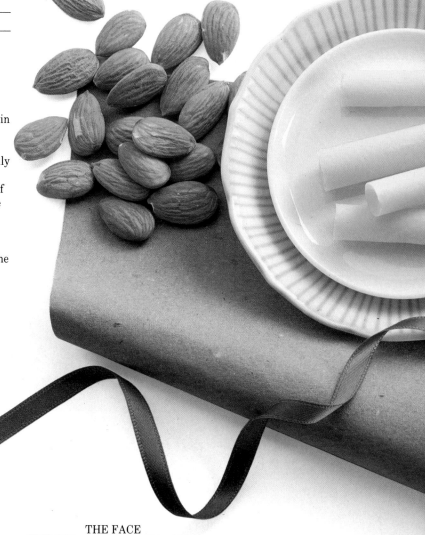

# Soothing mouthwash

*This helps protect the mucous membranes of the mouth, as it has antiseptic, astringent and healing properties.*

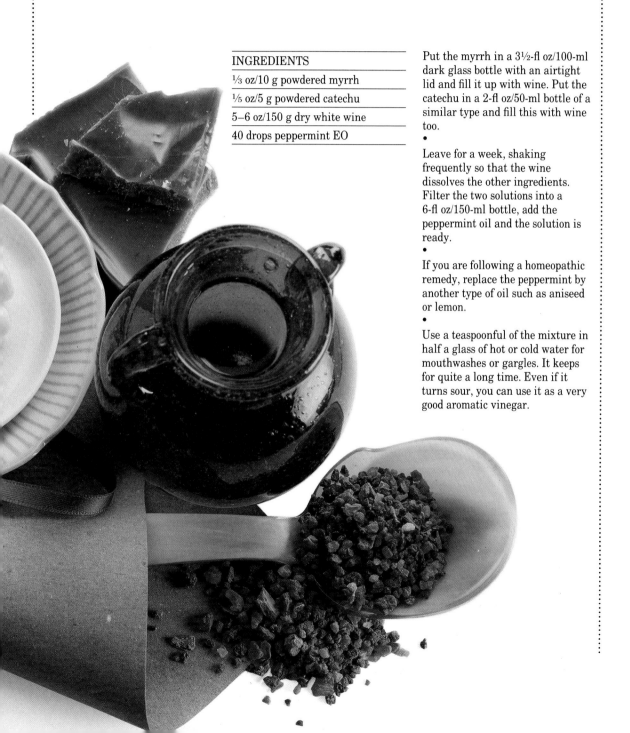

### INGREDIENTS

⅓ oz/10 g powdered myrrh

⅕ oz/5 g powdered catechu

5–6 oz/150 g dry white wine

40 drops peppermint EO

Put the myrrh in a 3½-fl oz/100-ml dark glass bottle with an airtight lid and fill it up with wine. Put the catechu in a 2-fl oz/50-ml bottle of a similar type and fill this with wine too.
•

Leave for a week, shaking frequently so that the wine dissolves the other ingredients. Filter the two solutions into a 6-fl oz/150-ml bottle, add the peppermint oil and the solution is ready.
•

If you are following a homeopathic remedy, replace the peppermint by another type of oil such as aniseed or lemon.
•

Use a teaspoonful of the mixture in half a glass of hot or cold water for mouthwashes or gargles. It keeps for quite a long time. Even if it turns sour, you can use it as a very good aromatic vinegar.

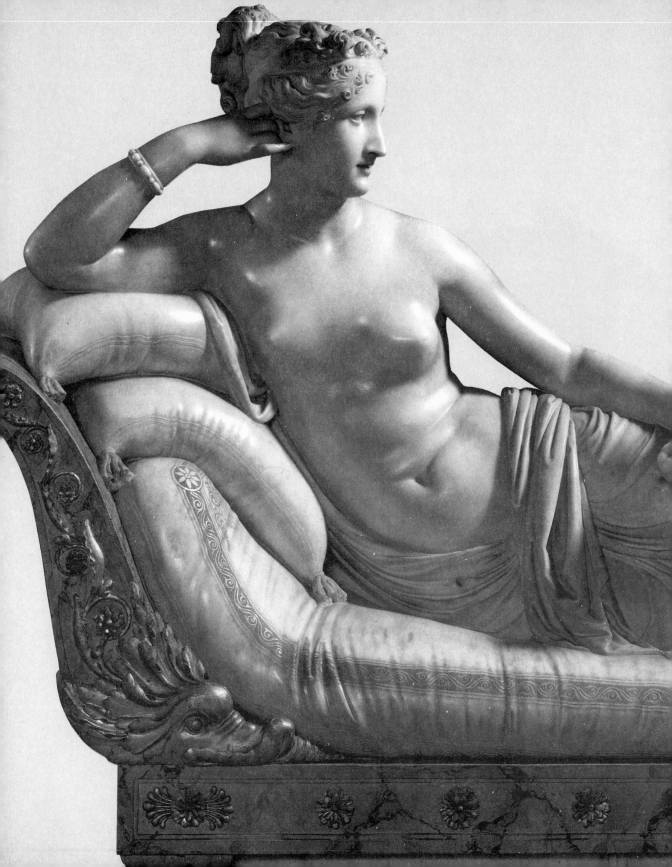

# The body

*Considerable importance is attached to personal hygiene nowadays, cleanliness being regarded as a prerequisite to good grooming. In previous eras, the emphasis was on the health-giving properties or medicinal value of the different substances used to cleanse the body. Also levels of hygiene and bathing customs have varied enormously, according to civilization and social classes. In this chapter you will find a collection of recipes from different periods and different countries.*

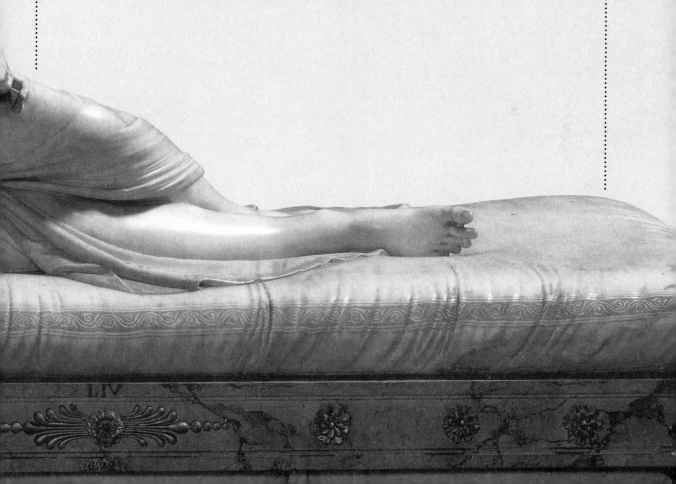

*In the past, it was mostly a privileged minority that could afford to spend time or money on body care. The following pages contain examples of the types of treatment that were used. The recipes have been modernized and some include exotic fruits now readily available that have proven cosmetic value. Some of the most basic body treatments were adopted by ordinary folk as well. For instance, the idea of cleaning the body using bran and flour mixed with water or other liquids was probably the result of discovering that kneading dough softened the hands. Even today, some people massage bread dough over their skin to deep-cleanse it. Clay or mud treatments fall under the same category, and oils have been used for cleansing since time immemorial in Mediterranean countries. "Handfuls" of oil, massaged over the body, plus a bucketful of water, were all that were needed by athletes to cleanse and smooth skin during training sessions. You will be amazed at how quickly you can regain a skin of childlike smoothness, once you stop drying it out with soap and lather. Try massaging yourself with almond oil for a few minutes and then taking a hot shower and rubbing yourself down with a cotton bag filled with 2–3 tablespoons of rice flour. You will notice an immediate improvement.*

# Massage oil

*It is incredible how thirsty our skin is for oil. For thousands of years, people have used oil on their skins as the only form of anti-wrinkle treatment.*

## INGREDIENTS

| |
|---|
| 3 tsp/15 g silver birch oil |
| 2 tsp/10 g horsetail oil |
| 3 tsp/15 g St. John's wort oil |
| 2 tsp/10 g stinging nettle oil |
| 3 tsp/15 g rose oil |
| 3 tsp/15 g elder oil |
| 2 tsp/10 g lime/linden oil |
| 20 drops rosemary EO |
| 50 drops lavender EO |

The oils should be obtained by maceration, ideally of fresh plants, according to the instructions at the beginning of the book. Pour them into a bottle and add the essential oils.

•

Shake thoroughly and massage the mixture over the body, a quarter of an hour before, or better still, after a shower, rubbing a few drops into the skin while it is wet and continuing until the oil has been fully absorbed.

•

If applying the oil to dry skin, it will be better absorbed if you wet your hands with water first.
Your skin will become soft and smooth, with a youthful bloom.

•

You can make up your own recipe, using two or more aromatic oils, according to the information in the charts and your personal tastes.

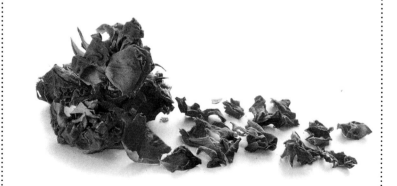

# Emollient body rub

*It is hard for us to accept that using familiar substances like soap or shower gel is not the only way of keeping clean. This unlikely cleansing mixture of fruit, cereals and herbs will leave your skin as soft and smooth as a child's.*

## INGREDIENTS

| |
| --- |
| 2 oz/50 g avocado flesh |
| 2 oz/50 g cucumber flesh |
| 2 oz/50 g lemon juice |
| 2 oz/50 g apple flesh |
| 2 oz/50 g whole milk natural yogurt |
| 1 tsp/5 g marigold oil |
| 1 tsp/5 g chamomile oil |
| 1 tsp/5 g wheatgerm oil |
| ⅓ oz/10 g green airfloat clay |
| 1 oz/25 g oat bran |
| 1 oz/25 g wholemeal soya flour |
| 50 drops lemon EO |

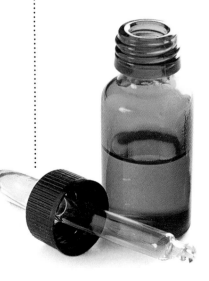

Weigh the ingredients carefully. Peel, clean and chop the avocado, cucumber and apple and put them in a blender. Add the lemon juice, yogurt and oil. Blend for a minute at low speed and a minute at high speed. Transfer the mixture to a plastic container and add the bran, flour and clay. Stir until thoroughly amalgamated.
•

Step into half a bathful of water and use the mixture to massage the body, leaving a thin layer on the skin so that the ingredients soak in.
•

The direction of massage will depend on which area you are treating: on the arms and legs use linear movements, from the extremities to the trunk; use mainly circular movements on the face and trunk. Do not hurry: massage yourself slowly and treat it as an opportunity to unwind.
•

Finally, sit down and soak for a few minutes. Then, rinse off all traces of the mixture with fresh lukewarm water.
•

If you can endure it, a final spray of cold water will stimulate circulation. Rub yourself vigorously with a soft towel, and the session is complete.
•

You can use mashed bananas instead of avocado. These are a bit less oily, so you may choose to double the quantity of one or more oils.

You can replace the oat bran with any type of cereal bran (wheat, barley, rye, etc.), but it must be finely milled. Similarly, you can use any type of legume flour (chick pea, pea, bean, etc.), although it should be wholemeal, to act as a gentle exfoliant. Leave out the essential oil or use a different type if you wish.
•

The mixture is sufficient for 1–2 treatments and can be kept refrigerated in an airtight container for 48 hours.

# Aromatic mud bath

*Every now and then, take a mud bath, using the special types
of clay which are available. They should be mixed until
creamy with an infusion of herbs.*

## INGREDIENTS

1 tbsp/2 g marigold flowers

1 tbsp/2 g lavender flowers

2–3 tbsp/2 g rose petals

⅓ oz/10 g powdered licorice root

2 tsp/10 g liquid honey

⅔ oz/20 g natural whole milk
  yogurt

1 tsp/4 g sweet almond oil

4 oz/120 g still mineral water

3½ oz/100 g clay

50 drops orange EO

Use the mixture described opposite
a little at a time (in dollops the size
of a walnut) to massage the whole
body, starting with the extremities
and working towards the center.
Use linear movements on the hands
and arms, feet and legs, and
circular straight movements
following the muscles on the face
and neck, chest and stomach.
•

Take your time: spend at least two
minutes on each part (two minutes
on the feet and ankles; two from the
ankles to knees, etc.). Leave a little
of the mixture on each area.
Finally, relax in the bath for 15–20
minutes while the mud and herbs

continue to act, even though
diluted.
•

Finish up with a shower, without
using any soap or other detergents.
Stroke away the mixture with the
hands and lukewarm water. Dry
yourself with a soft towel and then
wrap yourself naked in a wool
blanket and lie down to allow your
body to "react" (the mud, massage
and herbs will help rid the body of
toxins by inducing perspiration).

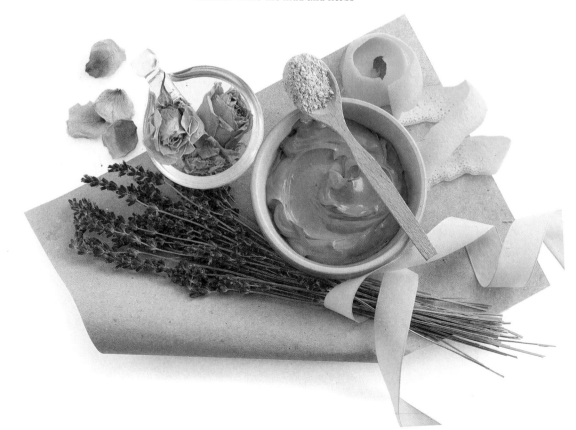

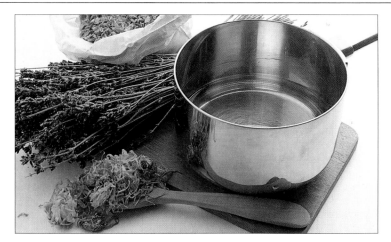

Weigh the ingredients carefully.

•

Boil the mineral water in a stainless
steel pan, then add the marigold and
lavender flowers and the rose petals.
Remove from the heat immediately
and cover.

•

Wait for 20 minutes, then strain the
infusion into a plastic bowl,
squeezing out the pulp.

•

Add the honey, yogurt, almond oil
and orange essential oil.

•

Dissolve the clay in this liquid, a
little at a time, stirring vigorously.
You may find it easier to use a hand
blender for this.

•

The amount of clay is purely
indicative. Different types will
absorb different amounts of water.

•

If your skin is very dry, you can
double the amount of almond oil.

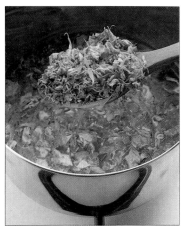
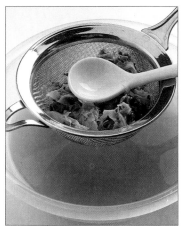

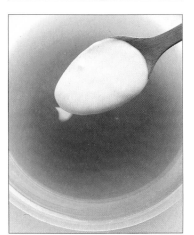
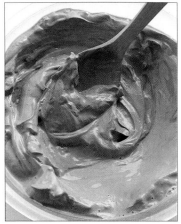

# Vegetable-protein skin smoothener

*This is a combination of abrasive and enzymatic exfoliation with an emollient herb treatment. It makes the skin wonderfully smooth.*

## INGREDIENTS

⅓ oz/10 g finely-milled oat bran

1 oz/30 g millet flour

⅔ oz/20 g ground almonds/almond meal

⅕ oz/5 g powdered licorice root

7 oz/200 g ripe pineapple flesh

2 tsp/10 g marigold oil

40 drops chamomile EO

lemon juice, as required

Skin the pineapple and cut the flesh into cubes. Blend these with the marigold oil and chamomile essential oil for a minute at low speed and a minute at high speed, until the mixture is smooth and creamy.

•

Add the bran a little at a time, then the ground almonds/almond meal and finally the millet flour, being careful not to make the mixture too stiff. The sound of the blender will tell you if it is getting too thick. Dilute with lemon juice if need be.

•

Massage the mixture on to the body, from the extremities inwards. Be gentle with the most delicate parts (face, breast) and more energetic on tougher areas like the feet, knees and elbows. Leave out the lips, eye area, nipples, etc., and areas with spots or any type of irritation. Leave a film of the mixture on the body as you go. Spend more time on rough skin like the feet and elbows. You should spend about 20–30 minutes in all.

•

Rinse under a lukewarm shower, without using soap or other detergents.

•

Rinsing is as important as the massage which preceded it. You must remove every trace of the mixture. Dry yourself carefully and your efforts will be rewarded by a soft, firm, young-looking skin.

•

This mixture works best if used immediately.

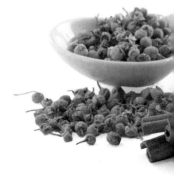

# Aromatic oil

*This refreshes and tones the body, relieves muscular tension
and leaves a spicy fragrance on the skin.*

## INGREDIENTS

| | |
|---|---|
| a pinch/2 g bay leaves (ground) | |
| ⅕ oz/5 g cinnamon | |
| ¹⁄₁₀ oz/3 g verbena leaves | |
| ¹⁄₁₀ oz/3 g cloves | |
| half pinch/1 g mace | |
| ¹⁄₁₀ oz/3 g marjoram leaves | |
| ⅕ oz/5 g chamomile flowers | |
| ¹⁄₁₀ oz/3 g rosemary leaves | |
| about ⅕ oz/4 g sage leaves | |
| a pinch/2 g thyme | |
| 50 drops lemon EO | |
| 14 oz/400 g still mineral water | |
| 1 oz/30 g horsetail stems | |
| 1 pint/½ liter brandy | |

Put the alcohol into an airtight, glass jar and add the first 11 ingredients. Leave to steep for two weeks, shaking the jar often, then strain through a paper filter into a 1½-pint/¾-liter bottle.

•

Make a decoction of horsetail stems by simmering them in the mineral water for 20 minutes.

Leave until lukewarm, then strain into the bottle with the herb mixture.

•

Massage the body with this oil occasionally after a bath, to relieve tired muscles and stiff joints.

•

Half a glassful can be added to bathwater; it can also be rubbed into the scalp, or even used as a mouthwash or gargle by adding a tablespoon to a glass of water.

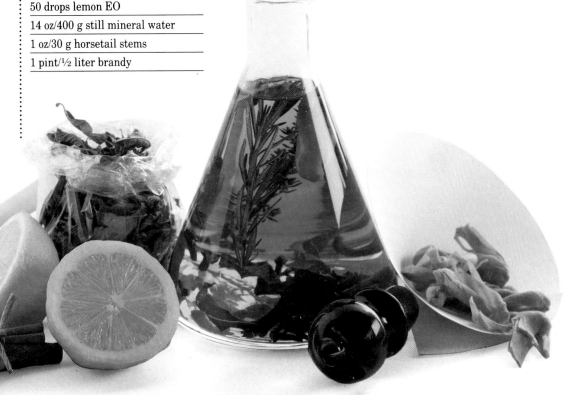

# Anti-cellulite poultice

*This is a useful complement to any type of cellulite treatment.*

## INGREDIENTS

1 tsp/5 g arnica oil

1 tsp/5 g ivy oil

1 tsp/5 g witch hazel oil

2 tsp/10 g horse-chestnut oil

1 tsp/5 g meadowsweet oil

2 tsp/10 g bladderwrack oil

50 drops rosemary EO

3½ oz/100 g linseed flour

14 oz/400 g still mineral water

Put the mineral water in a long-handled stainless steel pan and dissolve the linseed flour in this, over a gentle heat, stirring constantly until smooth.

•

Let it boil for a minute, then remove from the heat and add the oils. Stir again and pour a layer about ½ in/1 cm thick over a piece of muslin/cheesecloth large enough to leave a large edge around the poultice.

•

Fold the edges so that the poultice is closed like a packet. Check that it is not too hot by touching the smooth side against your palm, moistened with a few drops of oil. The temperature should be hot, but not scalding. You can prolong the heat by covering the poultice with a woollen blanket or hot water bottle.

•

Linseed flour soon spoils, so try to buy it freshly milled and vacuum-packed.

•

You can, if you wish, use a handful of fresh ivy leaves instead of ivy oil. After washing and drying them, chop them in a small blender and add them to the mixture.

Fresh ivy leaves can also be used in the bath, or as Dr. Leclerc, a famous French herbalist, suggested, they can be used to relieve neuritis and the skin discomfort which sometimes accompanies cellulite, as ivy reduces the sensitivity of the peripheral nerves.

•

This poultice could be used again the next day by adding a little water to reheat.

# Anti-cellulite cream

*This is a useful complement to cellulite treatments. Massage it in after exercising the muscles underlying the affected areas for at least 10 minutes.*

## INGREDIENTS

| |
|---|
| 2 tsp/10 g arnica oil |
| 2 tsp/10 g silver birch oil |
| 4 tsp/20 g ivy oil |
| 2 tsp/10 g fenugreek oil |
| 4 tsp/20 g horse-chestnut oil |
| 2 tsp/10 g bladderwrack oil |
| 2 tsp/10 g meadowsweet oil |
| 2¼ oz/60 g cocoa butter |
| ½ oz/15 g pure beeswax |
| 50 drops rosemary EO |

Weigh the ingredients carefully. Place the oils, cocoa butter and beeswax in a double boiler or stainless steel pan over a pan of water and dissolve to an oily liquid.

•

Replace the boiling water in the outer saucepan with cold and, using a hand blender, mix the oils thoroughly as they cool to a cream. Add the essential oil, mix again and put into clean, airtight jars. Keep refrigerated once the mixture has set. It will have a soft spreadable consistency.

•

The jar in use can be kept at room temperature. Massage small amounts into the skin from time to time, working upwards, towards the trunk.

•

The best massage would naturally be done by an expert. However, it is better to rub the cream in yourself, daily, than to have occasional treatments by a professional. You can always buy a book on massage if you wish to improve your technique.

•

Resist the temptation to use large amounts of cream. A little and often is the secret. You cannot expect results overnight, but if you persevere, you will win in the end.

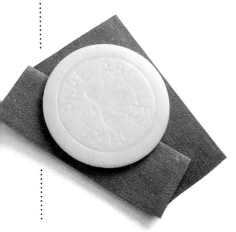

# Knee and elbow cream

*These are the parts of the body which are most neglected. This cream will give them some of the attention they deserve.*

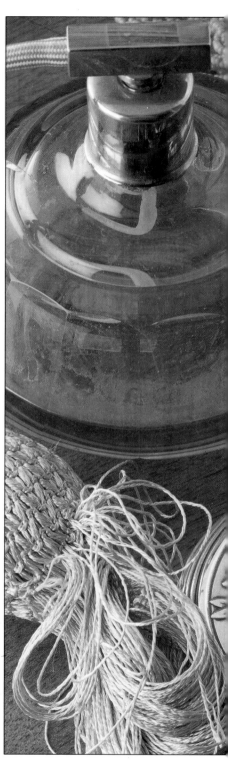

### INGREDIENTS

| |
|---|
| 4 tsp/20 g marigold oil |
| 2 tsp/10 g St. John's wort oil |
| 4 tsp/20 g chamomile oil |
| 1 oz/30 g cocoa butter |
| 1 oz/30 g diatomaceous earth |
| ⅓ oz/10 g chickpea flour |
| 1 drop orange EO |

Put the oils and cocoa butter in a double boiler and dissolve to a thick, oily liquid. Add the flour and earth and replace the water in the outer saucepan with cold. Stir vigorously until a cream is formed, then put into clean, airtight jars and refrigerate those not in use.
•

Gently massage small amounts into areas of rough skin such as the elbows, knees, soles of the feet or calloused hands. Do not rub too hard for too long as this cream is abrasive as well as softening. Rinse off with hot water.
A short treatment every day is better than the occasional, prolonged massage.
•

This cream is too abrasive to be used on the face or any areas that are easily irritated.

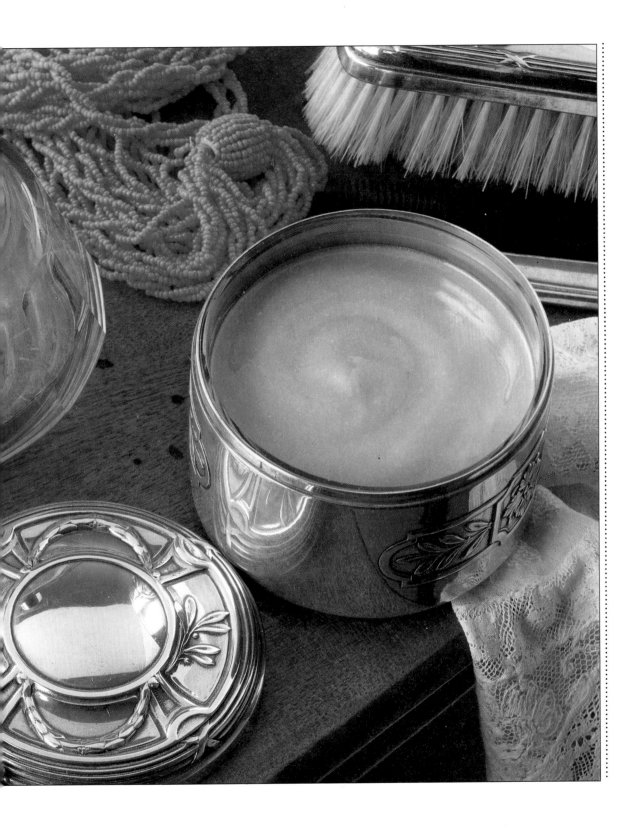

# Marsh mallow hand cream

*The hands are the part of the body most threatened by cold, burns, cuts and blisters. To keep them healthy and looking good, they need proper protection.*

### INGREDIENTS

| |
|---|
| 2 oz/50 g sweet almond oil |
| ²⁄₃ oz/20 g beeswax |
| ¹⁄₃ oz/10 g cocoa butter |
| ¹⁄₅ oz/5 g marsh mallow leaves |
| 5 oz/150 g still mineral water |
| 20 drops lemon EO |

Put the water and marsh mallow leaves in a stainless steel pan, bring to a boil and simmer for about 10 minutes, until nearly all the water has been absorbed.

•

When it is lukewarm, strain the decoction and put 1½ oz/40 g of the liquid back in the saucepan.
Melt the oil, wax and cocoa butter in a double boiler.

•

Reheat the marsh mallow juice almost to boiling and add it to the oily liquid a little at a time (if it were not hot, the oils would set). As you do so, mix it in with a hand blender, until a creamy emulsion is produced.

•

Put into clean, airtight jars and refrigerate.

This should be used as a barrier cream before and after "dry" domestic chores. If you are doing "wet" housework (e.g. hand washing clothes or dishes) or jobs which involve contact with chemicals (e.g. cleaning silver), spread plenty of cream on the hands, protect them with cotton gloves, and then put a pair of rubber gloves on top.

•

For perfect hands, use a little of this cream each time you wash and dry them. It will replace the natural moisture which protects the skin

•

The jar in use need not be refrigerated.

# Almond hand-washing paste

*If the eyes are the mirror of the soul, the hands reflect our lifestyle: the type of work we do, and possibly even our character. We should treat them properly.*

### INGREDIENTS

2 oz/50 g ground almonds/almond meal

4 tsp/20 g almond oil

4 tsp/20 g lemon juice

1½ oz/40 g brandy

Mix the ingredients gently in a mortar. If you do not have a pestle and mortar, a fork and dish will do. Work the ingredients together, as you would to prepare stuffing.

•

Fill airtight jars with the mixture and keep what you are not using refrigerated. Use a quantity the size of a walnut, in the same way as soap. Rinse off carefully.

•

Detergents, cold weather and overwashing roughen and crack the skin. With regular use, this paste will rectify the problem, softening the hands as well as cleaning them.

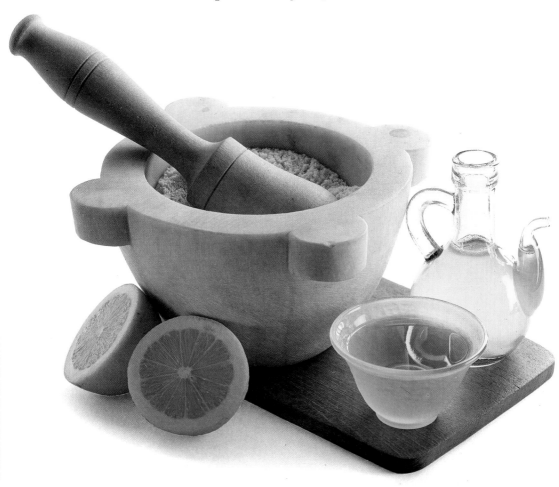

# Hand-washing powder

*This cleans the hands and makes them soft and smooth. It is especially good for people whose hands are always in water.*

## INGREDIENTS

1½ oz/40 g ground almonds/almond meal

⅓ oz/10 g rice flour

⅓ oz/10 g powdered orris root

2 tsp/10 g sweet almond oil

50 drops lavender or lemon EO

Put the almonds and almond oil in a mortar or bowl. Mix vigorously with pestle or spoon until the oil is absorbed. You can use a blender for this if you wish, running it briefly at low speed.
Add the rice flour, orris root and lavender EO and mix again.

•

Use a pinch of the mixture on wet hands, in the same way as soap.

•

If you prefer, you can turn the powder into a paste by adding ⅔ oz/20 g anhydrous glycerine and mixing thoroughly.

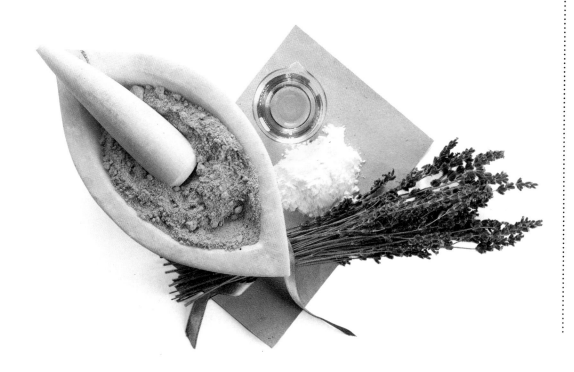

# The Queen of Hungary's toilet water

*This toilet water is based on a recipe from the fourteenth century, which was said to have been responsible for the good health and youthful appearance of the seventy-year-old sovereign.*

### INGREDIENTS

1 oz/30 g rosemary flowering heads

⅓ oz/10 g lavender flowers

⅓ oz/10 g juniper leaves

¾ tsp/3 g purified EO of camphor

1 pint/½ liter dry white wine

Steep the ingredients in the white wine for a week in an airtight jar. Shake daily.

•

Strain the mixture and store the liquid in airtight, dark glass jars in a cool, dark place.

•

Use as an occasional skin toner on the face and body, as a hair lotion between shampoos, or as a refreshing addition to bathwater.

•

Naturally, there are no guarantees that this recipe will take years off your age, but it will do no harm and is easy to make.
The Queen of Hungary had a court alchemist at her disposal. Who knows what other ingredients may have been added to the mixture!

•

Rosemary is very good for the skin and hair. It is a sun-loving plant and has a wonderful aroma. Originally a Mediterranean plant, it grows well in open, sunny places. Lavender thrives in both dry, sunny areas and damp climates. Its flowers are full of essential oil.

# Foot cream

*After a bath, treat your feet to this cream.*
*It soothes, tired, swollen feet, ankles and calves.*

INGREDIENTS

| | |
|---|---|
| 2 tsp/10 g marigold oil | ½ oz/15 g kaolin |
| 2 tsp/10 g lavender oil | ⅕ oz/5 g rice flour |
| 4 tsp/20 g rosemary oil | 40 drops lavender EO |
| 2 tsp/10 g sage oil | ⅕ oz/5 g bay leaves |
| 2 tsp/10 g wine tincture of catechu | 3½ oz/100 g still mineral water |
| 50 drops tincture of propolis | ½ oz/15 g pure beeswax |
| | ½ oz/15 g cocoa butter |

Prepare the cream according to the instructions opposite and store the jars in the refrigerator.

•

It will keep better if you put a drop of EO of lavender on the surface of each jar of cream before closing it up.

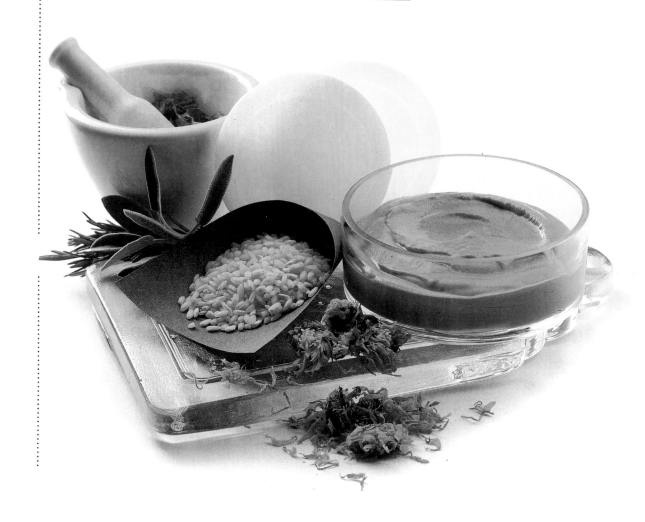

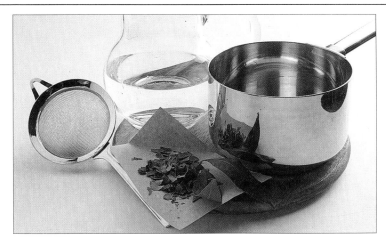

Measure out the herbs carefully.

•

Bring the mineral water to a boil and add the chopped bay leaves. Remove from heat and after 20 minutes strain the mixture, putting the liquid back in the pan.

•

Add the catechu, kaolin, rice flour and propolis drops, stirring constantly over a very low heat, until the mixture forms a gel. You can use a spoon or a hand blender. Leave with the lid on.

•

Melt the beeswax, cocoa butter and marigold, lavender, rosemary and sage oils in a double boiler. When they are thoroughly blended, add the gel mixture a little at a time, combining them with a hand blender. Replace the boiling water of the outer saucepan with cold and, still mixing, add the essential oil of lavender. The cream will thicken as it cools and should then be put into clean, airtight jars.

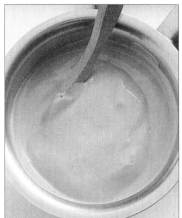

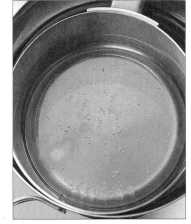

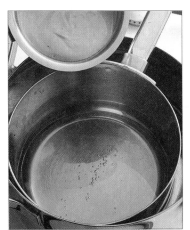

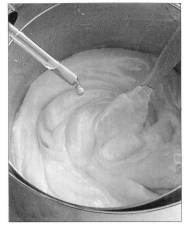

# Soothing footbath

*The feet have to bear the weight of the whole body, so it is hardly surprising that they become tired and painful. You should look after them.*

### INGREDIENTS

⅓ oz/10 g bay leaves

⅕ oz/5 g lavender flowers

⅓ oz/10 g marsh mallow leaves

⅕ oz/5 g walnut leaves

⅓ oz/10 g rosemary leaves

⅓ oz/10 g sage leaves

4 pints/2 liters still mineral water

Heat the water in a stainless steel pan and add the herbs as soon as it boils. Remove from the heat immediately and cover.

•

Wait for 15 minutes, then strain the infusion into a large bowl.

•

If your feet tend to perspire, you can add 10 drops of essential oil of thyme to the footbath.

•

Immerse your feet for at least 15 minutes, keeping the temperature of the infusion constant by adding more hot water. Dry them carefully and dust with a foot powder or massage with a foot cream if desired.

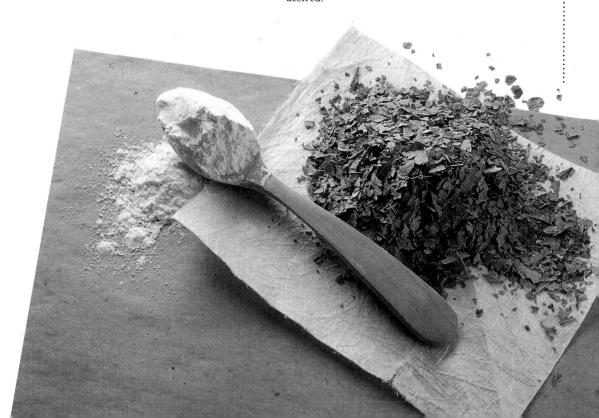

# Kaolin foot powder

*This is a foot powder for those who exercise frequently, wear sports footwear much of the time, or for whom sweaty feet are a real problem.*

### INGREDIENTS

3½ oz/100 g kaolin

1 oz/30 g rice flour

1 oz/30 g club moss spores

about 1 oz/25 g elder leaves

about 1 oz/25 g sage leaves

50 drops peppermint EO

30 drops thyme EO

Put the sage and elder leaves in a blender and run it for a minute at low speed and a minute at high speed. Using a fine, mesh sieve, strain the resulting powder two tablespoons at a time and use only the finest part.

•

Put all the ingredients in a bottle, jar or plastic container and shake them. Add the essential oil using a dropper and shake the mixture as you go.

•

Massage small quantities into the feet, or dust socks or shoes with it. You should wear only cotton or wool socks and leather shoes, rope sandals or wooden clogs.

•

The powder will keep well at room temperature.

•

The *flowers* of the elder, on the other hand, have a beneficial effect on sore skin. Collect and dry them in the shade and store them in an airtight container in the dark. An infusion makes a soothing, emollient compress for inflamed skin and sore eyes.

# Deodorant

*The best deodorant is thorough washing every day, but if this is not enough . . .*

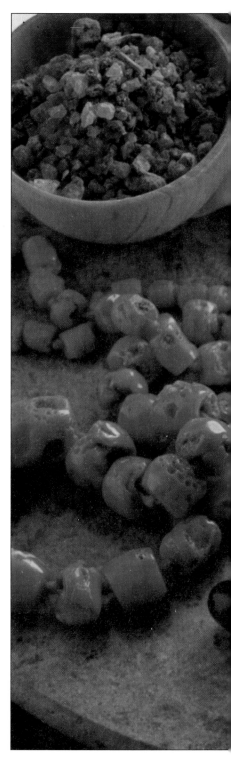

## INGREDIENTS

| |
|---|
| ⅓ oz/8 g tincture of myrrh |
| about ⅕ oz/4 g tincture of catechu |
| 5 oz/150 g dry white wine |
| 20 drops lavender EO |
| 50 drops lemon EO |
| 5 drops clove EO |
| 50 drops marigold EO |

Pour all the ingredients into a bottle and shake to mix. Put a little on a piece of cotton wool/cotton and apply to freshly washed and dried skin. It can also be used on the feet.

•

The best substances for washing the skin before you use this are water and starch (corn flour, rice flour), possibly with the addition of a few drops of essential oil and some diluted cider vinegar. These are completely harmless and you need have no qualms about using them. Do not get carried away with quantities and end up smelling of disinfectant, rather than just fresh and clean.

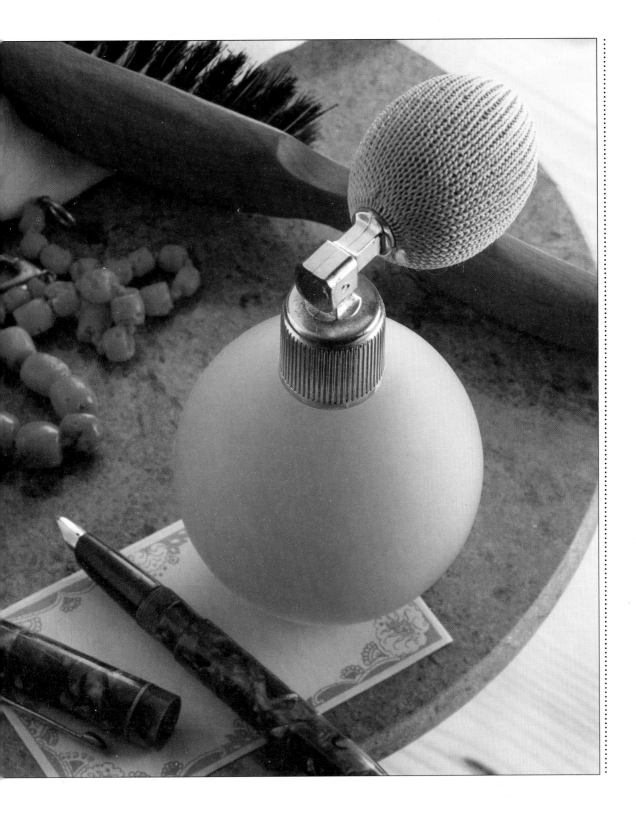

# Intimate deodorant

*This is a gentle deodorant and astringent: a useful aid to female personal hygiene.*

## INGREDIENTS

2 tsp/10 g tincture of benzoin

2 tsp/10 g tincture of myrrh

1 tsp/5 g tincture of cinchona

½ oz/15 g rice flour

3½ oz/100 g cider vinegar

⅕ oz/5 g Iceland moss

7 oz/200 g still mineral water

50 drops marigold EO

50 drops lavender EO

20 drops lemon EO

Put the water and Iceland moss in a stainless steel pan. Bring to a boil very slowly and simmer for 15 minutes. Remove from the heat and cover. When lukewarm, strain into a bottle and add the other ingredients.

•

Shake the bottle before using the mixture. Use a tablespoon for every 4 pints/2 liters of water in the bidet or bath.

•

The mixture will keep at room temperature.

•

A different version can be made for men, by replacing the essential oils with:
5 drops clove EO
25 drops lemon EO
90 drops sandalwood EO

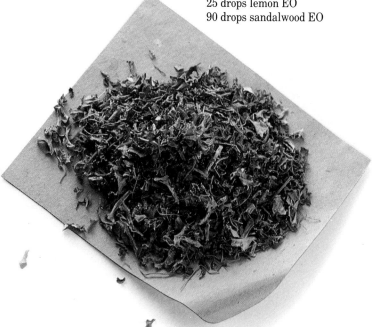

# Salt water bath

*Bathing in warm salt water, sometimes with seaweed, has been practiced throughout the world since antiquity. It acts as a tonic.*

### INGREDIENTS

2¼ lb/1 kg unbleached sea salt

13 gallons/50 liters water

optional extras:

2 oz/50 g powdered bladderwrack

4½ lb/2 kg still mineral water

Put the salt in the bath, keeping the ratio of salt to water 2¼ lb/1 kg salt : 13 gallons/50 liters water. The water should be a little warmer than body temperature (100°F/37.5°C).

•

The easiest way of measuring the water is to fill a large 2-gallon or 10-liter jug, bowl or bucket and empty it into the bathtub as needed. Then measure the depth of the water by holding a ruler vertically over the plug (the average depth will be about 5 in/12 cm). That way, you will know how much water to use next time.

•

Sit in the bath for 15–20 minutes, massaging yourself gently with a natural sponge, so that the whole body benefits from contact with the saline solution.

•

Tepid salt water is a great tonic. It is good for rheumatism and allergies, and has an anti-inflammatory action against many types of gynecological problems. Obviously you should seek medical advice as well when symptoms appear.

•

The amount of salt suggested in the recipe is far less than the natural salinity of seawater, but enough for cosmetic purposes.

•

After 15–20 minutes, dry yourself briskly, without rinsing off the water, so that the salt can continue to act. Then wrap yourself naked in a wool blanket and lie down to allow your body to react by expelling toxins in the form of perspiration. After about half an hour, take a warm shower of water only, to remove the salt and impurities.

•

You can turn this into a treatment for cellulite by adding the mineral water and bladderwrack. These should be simmered in a stainless steel pan for 15 minutes, left to cool for another 15 minutes and then strained into the bathtub. Then proceed as for the other bath.

# Emollient bath

*This smooths the skin and tones the muscles and is ideal
after strenuous exercise or a tiring day.*

## INGREDIENTS

⅓ oz/10 g yarrow flower heads

⅓ oz/10 g marigold flowers

⅓ oz/10 g chamomile flowers

⅓ oz/10 g helichrysum (everlasting)
  flowers

⅔ oz/20 g lavender flowers

⅓ oz/10 g red rose flowers

⅓ oz/10 g rosemary leaves

⅓ oz/10 g sage leaves

6 pints/3 liters still mineral water

7 oz/200 g wheat bran

2 oz/50 g rice flour

2 tsp/10 g sweet almond oil

Take a relaxing bath for at least 20
minutes, using the mixture
described opposite, and massage
your body gently with the bag of
bran. Do not use soap or other
detergents. Your skin will feel
wonderful afterwards, as this bath
softens and refines the skin and
stimulates the circulation.

You can finish with a heat
treatment: dry vigorously, then
wrap yourself in a wool blanket and
lie down for half an hour. Your body
will eliminate toxins through gentle
perspiration.

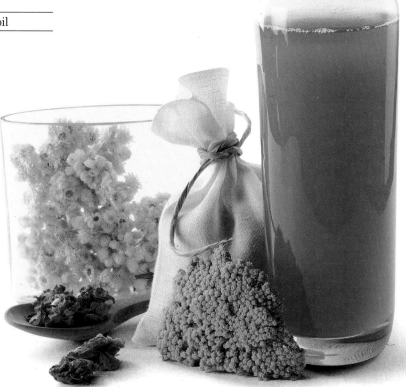

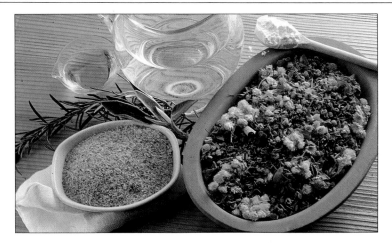

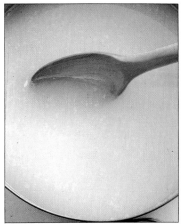

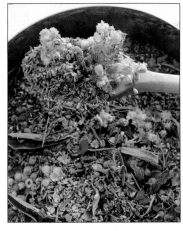

*Measure out the ingredients carefully.*

•

*Put the water and rice flour in a stainless steel pan away from the heat and stir until the mixture is free of lumps. Bring to the boil, stirring constantly to prevent it sticking to the bottom.*

•

*As soon as it boils, add the herbs, remove from the heat and cover. Let steep for at least 15 minutes.*

•

*Meanwhile, put the bran in a muslin/cheesecloth bag and tie the top with string. Protecting your hands with gloves, hold the bag under the hot water tap in the bath squeezing and wringing it out like a sponge, so that the bran releases its active principles into the bath water which will look like a milky solution. Mix with cold water until the bathwater is the right temperature.*

•

*Add the almond oil and stir it around with one hand. The bath will not make your body greasy. The almond oil will be distributed over the surface of the skin, helping the emollient action of the starch in the flour and bran to make your skin smoother, more elastic and younger looking.*

*When the infusion is ready strain it through a colander into the water and then the bath will be ready.*

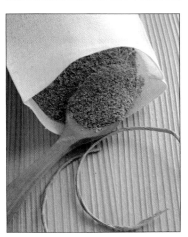

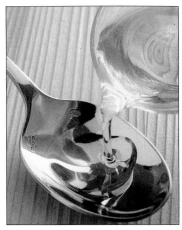

# Balsamic toning bath

*This is recommended for sportsmen and women. It is particularly good for lungs and bronchial tubes.*

### INGREDIENTS

⅓ oz/10 g silver fir leaves

⅓ oz/10 g bay leaves

⅓ oz/10 g eucalyptus leaves

⅓ oz/10 g juniper leaves

⅓ oz/10 g marjoram leaves

⅓ oz/10 g peppermint leaves

⅓ oz/10 g Swiss mountain pine buds (crushed)

⅓ oz/10 g rosemary leaves

⅓ oz/10 g thyme leaves

2 oz/50 g rice flour

2 tsp/10 g sweet almond oil

6 pints/3 liters still mineral water

Beat the rice flour into the water in a large stainless steel pan away from the heat, then bring it gently to a boil, stirring constantly. Add the herbs, remove from the heat and cover.

•

Wait for 15 minutes, during which time you can run the bath and add the almond oil, stirring it round to disperse the droplets of oil.

•

Strain the herb liquid into the bath.

•

Take a 15–20 minute bath, rubbing yourself vigorously with a sponge (not a loofah).

•

Do not use soap or other detergents: the rice flour will cleanse the body perfectly well.

# Sedative bath

*This is very good for adults or children who are highly strung and need to relax before going to bed in order to sleep.*

## INGREDIENTS

| |
|---|
| ⅕ oz/5 g yarrow flower heads |
| ⅓ oz/10 g orange leaves |
| ⅕ oz/5 g marigold flowers |
| ⅓ oz/10 g chamomile flowers |
| ⅓ oz/10 g lemon leaves |
| ⅓ oz/10 g lemon balm flower heads |
| ⅓ oz/10 g peppermint leaves |
| ⅓ oz/10 g (field) poppy petals |
| ⅓ oz/10 g lime/linden flowers |
| ⅓ oz/10 g lemon verbena leaves |
| 5 oz/150 g oat bran |
| 6 pints/3 liters still mineral water |

Put the water and bran in a large stainless steel pan. Bring to a boil and simmer for 5 minutes. Add the herbs, remove from the heat and cover. Wait for 15 minutes, during which time you can run the bath (suggested temperature: 100°F/37.5°C). Strain the contents of the saucepan into the bath, through a muslin/cheesecloth bag, so that the solid parts are left inside the bag, which should then be closed with string.

Use the bag like a washcloth to massage yourself as you bathe. Do not use soap or other detergents. After this bath, you will be ready to go to bed and fall into a deep sleep. The bag can also be made from a piece of cotton, hemmed around three sides in a U-shape.

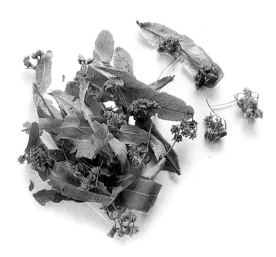

# Classical bath

*This is a humbler edition of the famous bath in "asses' milk" which Poppea, wife of Nero, used to indulge in.*

## INGREDIENTS

4 pints/2 liters whole cow's milk

2 oz/50 g liquid acacia honey

2 oz/50 g tincture of benzoin

30 drops orange EO

10 drops cinnamon EO

5 drops clove EO

10 drops lemon EO

Pour the ingredients into the bathtub, together with the hot water. Steep a natural sponge in the liquid and massage your body, so that the emollient substances in the milk and the essential oils can take effect. Do not use soap. Add 5 drops of sandalwood essential oil for extra fragrance.

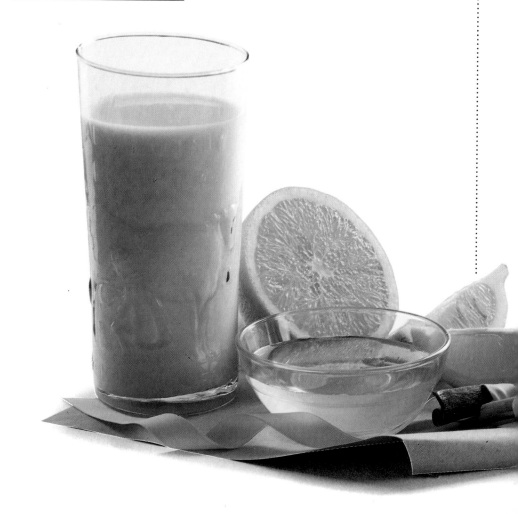

# Aromatic baths

*These baths are like an oasis in the desert for weary travellers or for people who lead busy lives.*

### INGREDIENTS: SPICY CITRUS BATH

| | |
|---|---|
| 1 tsp/5 ml Seville orange EO | |
| ½ tsp/3 ml cinnamon EO | |
| 1 tsp/5 ml lemon verbena EO | |
| ¼ tsp/2 ml coriander EO | |
| ¼ tsp/2 ml clove EO | |
| ½ tsp/3 ml sage EO | |
| 1 tsp/5 ml sandalwood EO | |
| 8 oz/250 g tincture of benzoin | |
| 4 tsp/20 g avocado oil | |

### INGREDIENTS: WOODLAND BATH

| | |
|---|---|
| 1 tsp/5 ml green aniseed EO | |
| ½ tsp/3 ml basil EO | |
| ¼ tsp/2 ml Mediterranean cypress EO | |
| ¼ tsp/2 ml eucalyptus EO | |
| 1 tsp/5 ml peppermint EO | |
| ½ tsp/3 ml Swiss mountain pine EO | |

| | |
|---|---|
| 1 tsp/5 ml rosemary EO | |
| 8 oz/250 g tincture myrrh | |
| 4 tsp/20 g avocado oil | |

For either recipe, put the ingredients into an airtight jar and shake to mix. Shake also before each use. Add one tablespoonful to your bathwater to make an aromatic bath.

•

You can vary the essential oils to suit yourself. They have a refreshing effect, as they penetrate the skin and stimulate the circulation. According to aromatherapists, these perfumes also influence one's state of mind, and can be used to relieve stress or improve a person's outlook.

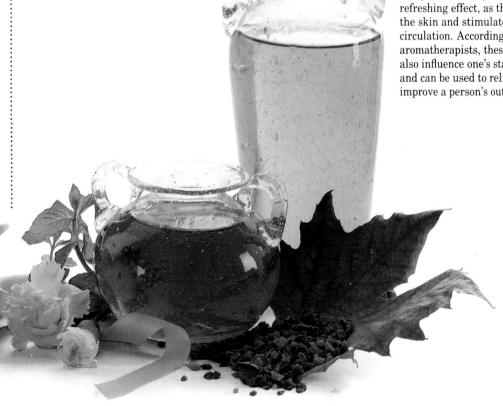

# Body cream

*This can be added to bathwater or massaged over the body, undiluted, with a sponge. It leaves the skin smooth, elastic and fragrant.*

### INGREDIENTS

2 oz/60 g marsh mallow root

about 2 oz/50 g white bread, without crust

3 pints/1½ liters still mineral water

1¼ oz/35 g cream

1 egg yolk

2 tbsp/30 g tincture of myrrh

4 tsp/20 g tincture of benzoin

Break up the marsh mallow root, crumble the bread and boil them in the mineral water for 20 minutes, stirring occasionally.
Strain them into a bottle, add the egg yolk, cream and tinctures, and shake thoroughly.
This keeps for a week in the refrigerator.

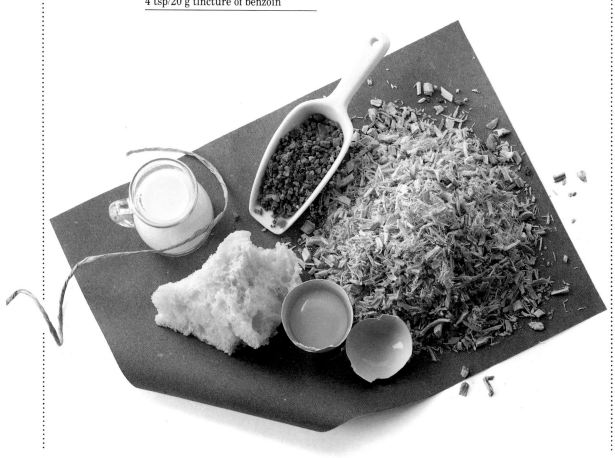

# SUNSCREENS AND TANNING COSMETICS

*It is now an established fact that, if people gave up sunbathing, the number of patients with skin problems would be reduced by at least a quarter.*

*The sun is in fact the main cause of skin ageing apart from the process of growing old. You only need to look at the face of an old seafarer, farmer or mountain-dweller from the Mediterranean countries to be convinced of this. His face will be a mass of wrinkles on a skin as dry as parchment, at least 10–15 years before it should be. Conversely, those who live in the north – where it is often cloudy and the sun is less strong – frequently look a great deal younger than they are. This is borne out by past experience, when women used to avoid the sun, in the firm belief that the whiter their skin, the better they would look. The fashion was taken to the point where, in the last century, ruddy-cheeked countrywomen did untold damage to their health in an effort to achieve the pale, "aristocratic" complexion that was all the rage. They would drink glassfuls of vinegar, which caused anaemia and gastric ulcers. With the same lack of foresight, their great-grandchildren spend hours roasting in the sun for a fashionable golden tan.*

*This is not to say that the sun is entirely harmful. Spending time in warm sunshine can be beneficial in terms of both mental and physical health – it is without doubt good for the morale. But you should limit sun exposure, especially when you are not used to it. Remember that when on the beach, even if you stay under an umbrella, the sand and water reflect the sun's ultraviolet rays, so that time in the shade should be included when calculating your sun exposure. The only real protection is light clothing, plus a wide-brimmed hat of the type worn by our great-grandmothers, who knew what they were doing. The length of time you can afford to spend in the sun will depend on how sensitive your skin is, what type of colouring you have, and the time of day. The sun reaches its maximum intensity during the 3–4 hours around midday, and you will need to be particularly careful during the first few days of your holiday. Resist the temptation to acquire a tan as fast as possible, use high-factor sun creams, and step up your exposure time gradually, particularly if you are holidaying in the deep south. People with blue eyes, red hair and pale skin are the most at risk. If you burn your skin, this prevents it from going brown and you will pay for such maltreatment in later years. Prevention is better than cure. Therefore, a month before going on a holiday by the sea or in the mountains, eat plenty of foods full of vitamins. Citrus fruits, and raw vegetables like carrots, cabbage and spinach, help the body to produce plenty of melanin, the dark pigment which is responsible for tanning. You can also add food supplements to your diet, like wheatgerm, brewer's yeast and pollen. These are available from pharmacies, herbalists and supermarkets. Take them together in small doses, so that your body will have a whole range of vitamins, aminoacids, mineral salts and trace elements to help cope with the tanning process.*

*Remember that some medicines make the skin photosensitive or are harmful if you sunbathe while taking them. These include some oral contraceptives, several forms of antibiotic, sulfa drugs, some diuretics and cortisones, some artificial sweeteners and vegetable-based laxatives, and some antihistamines and tranquillizers. If you are taking medicines, check first.*

*Keep in mind that essential oils from citrus fruits, rue, fennel and angelica can contain substances which cause indelible pigment changes if you sunbathe for long after using them. The same applies to a number of perfumes, which are a mixture of essential oils; avoid using them when you are going out to sunbathe as the body marks remain. Finally remember that it is a good idea to help your skin on days you are sunbathing by taking soothing, emollient baths.*

# Suntan cream

*This is an excellent suntan lotion. It does not contain any suntan block so use your common sense and do not stay in the sun for too long.*

## INGREDIENTS

2 tsp/10 g avocado oil

4 tsp/20 g jojoba oil

2 tsp/10 g castor oil

4 tsp/20 g sesame oil

1 oz/30 g cocoa butter

1/3 oz/10 g shea butter

1/3 oz/10 g pure beeswax

2 tsp/10 g marigold oil

2 tsp/10 g St. John's wort oil

2/3 oz/20 g walnut husk oil

1 tsp/2 g powdered aloe vera

2 oz/50 g still mineral water

3/4 tsp/2 g soya lecithin

Melt the oils, butters and wax in a double boiler over a gentle heat, until they are reduced to an oily liquid. If using liquid soya lecithin, add it to the oils. If using granules, dissolve them in the mineral water, together with the powdered aloe vera, using a double boiler or a container over a pan of hot water. Strain this last mixture into the pan of fats and oils.
•

Replace the boiling water in the outer saucepan with cold and, using a hand blender, mix the ingredients together. They will form a cream as they cool. Put this into clean, airtight jars and keep all but the one in use in the refrigerator.
•

Aloe vera gives the skin a bitter taste: leave the ingredient out if this bothers you.

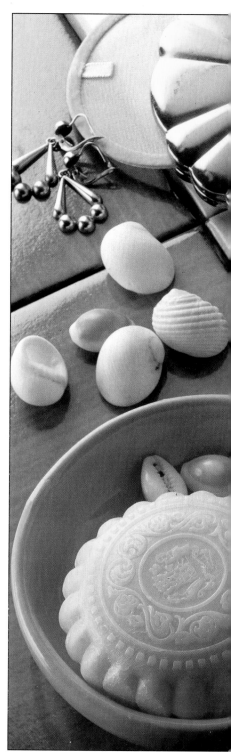

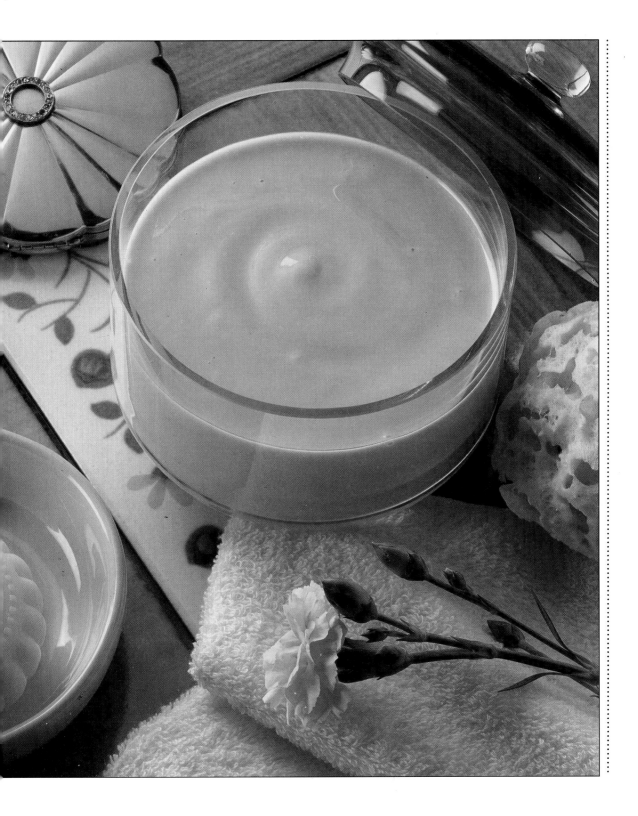

# Suntan oil

*Natural sunscreens do have a limited filtering ability, but this is one of the best.*

## INGREDIENTS

| |
|---|
| 2 tsp/10 g avocado oil |
| 4 tsp/20 g jojoba oil |
| 2 tsp/10 g castor oil |
| 4 tsp/20 g sesame oil |
| ⅓ oz/10 g shea butter |
| 2 tsp/10 g marigold oil |
| 2 tsp/10 g St. John's wort oil |
| 2 tsp/10 g walnut husk oil |

Mix the avocado, jojoba, castor and sesame oils with the shea butter in a double boiler, or stainless steel pan over a pan of water, and heat gently. Using a hand blender, mix until smooth.

•

Pour into an airtight, dark glass bottle, together with the marigold, St. John's wort and walnut husk oils. Shake the bottle.

•

Make your own marigold, St. John's wort and walnut husk oils with a base of extra-virgin olive oil to make the recipe even better.

Massage a little of the mixture into the skin before sunbathing, paying particular attention to the face, shoulders, chest, stomach and fronts of the thighs, which are the parts most likely to burn. Repeat this massage several times, after bathing, or vigorous exercise. If you perspire, do not wipe off the moisture: it contains natural body substances which help prevent sunburn.

•

This oil will keep perfectly well for the length of time of your holiday.

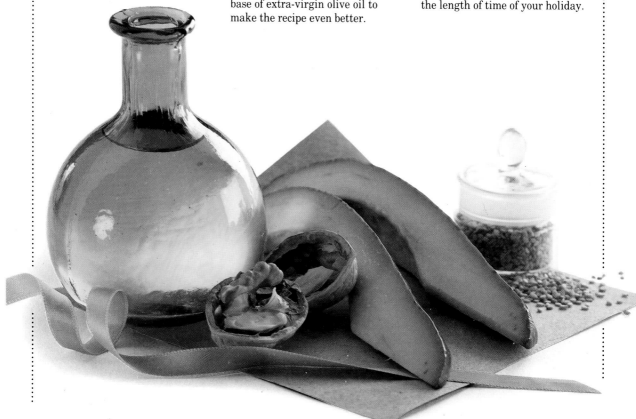

# Aftersun cream

*This has many of the same ingredients as the lotion overleaf, but because it is a cream, it is better for use after winter sports.*

## INGREDIENTS

1 tsp/5 g avocado oil

1 tsp/5 g castor oil

⅔ oz/20 g cocoa butter

⅓ oz/10 g shea butter

1 tsp/5 g chamomile oil

1 tsp/5 g helichrysum (everlasting) oil

1 tsp/5 g St. John's wort oil

⅓ oz/10 g pure beeswax

⅓ oz/10 g marsh mallow root

⅓ oz/10 g powdered licorice root

½ oz/15 g kaolin

8 oz/220 g still mineral water

Chop the marsh mallow root as small as possible and add to the water and licorice root in a stainless steel pan.
Bring to a boil and simmer for 10 minutes. Remove from the heat, cover and let steep for 15 minutes.
•
Melt the oils, fats and wax in a double boiler.
•
Strain the marsh mallow and licorice decoction into a bowl, add the kaolin and mix to a smooth consistency.
Pour the mixture a little at a time into the pan of oils and mix with a hand blender. Replace the hot water in the double saucepan with cold and blend the ingredients until creamy.
Transfer the cream to clean, airtight jars and refrigerate to set.

# Aftersun lotion

*This moisturizing lotion is anti-inflammatory and reduces redness.*

## INGREDIENTS

| |
|---|
| 1 tsp/5 g avocado oil |
| 1 tsp/5 g castor oil |
| ⅓ oz/10 g cocoa butter |
| ⅓ oz/10 g shea butter |
| 1 tsp/5 g chamomile oil |
| 1 tsp/5 g helichrysum (everlasting) oil |
| 1 tsp/5 g St. John's wort oil |
| ¾ tsp/2 g soya lecithin |
| ½ tsp/1 g white clay |
| 1 tsp/2 g powdered aloe vera |
| ⅓ oz/10 g powdered licorice root |
| ⅓ oz/10 g butcher's broom root |
| ⅓ oz/10 g marsh mallow leaves |
| 5 oz/150 g dry white wine |
| 8 oz/220 g still mineral water |

The lotion described opposite is very good after a shower or an emollient bath. It should be massaged over the whole body, concentrating on areas that have been exposed to the sun.

Aloe vera gives the skin a bitter taste: if you do not like it, add a tablespoon of cider vinegar instead. The mixture keeps for 7–10 days refrigerated.

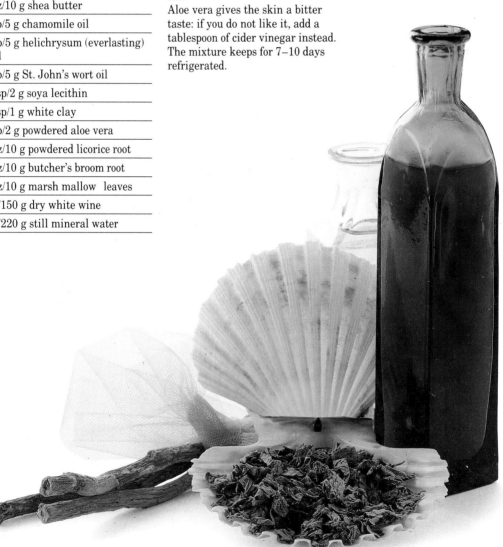

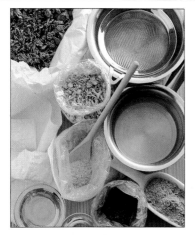

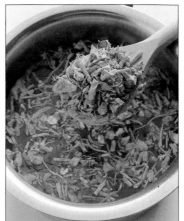

*Weigh the herbs carefully.*

•

*Chop the butcher's broom as small as possible and place it and the wine in a saucepan.*

•

*Bring to a boil and simmer for 5 minutes. Remove from the heat, cover and let steep for 15 minutes. Put the water, marsh mallow leaves and licorice root in another saucepan. Bring to a boil and simmer for 10 minutes. Remove from the heat. Add the aloe vera, stir, cover and leave for 15 minutes.*

•

*Strain the two mixtures into a third saucepan, squeezing out the herbs. Add the white clay and soya lecithin and dissolve them over a very gentle heat, stirring constantly until the mixture forms a gel.*
*Using a double boiler, melt the cocoa and shea butter in the oils. Add the contents of the third saucepan and mix with a hand blender.*

•

*Replace the hot water in the outer saucepan with cold. Give the lotion a final whisk as it cools and place in airtight, dark glass bottles, which should be kept refrigerated when not in use.*
*Shake well before use.*

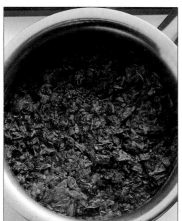

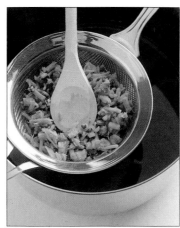

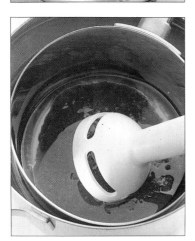

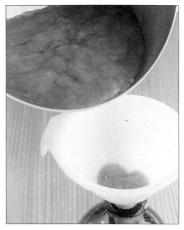

# Glossary

**Acne.** An inflammatory disorder of the sebaceous glands, caused by a blockage and resulting in spots and pimples. Normally occurs during adolescence when hormonal levels rise at puberty.

**Antiseptic.** Destroys the microorganisms that cause infection.

**Astringent.** A substance that tightens the pores. Alcohol is often used as an antiseptic astringent but it has a strong, very drying effect. Milder, more soothing astringents are rosewater and almond meal. Astringents are usually used to clean oily skins.

**Decoction.** A method of extracting the water-soluble active ingredients of herbs and other plant parts. The herbs are boiled in water and the extract used internally or externally for medicinal and cosmetic purposes.

**Disinfectant.** A substance that eliminates or prevents the growth of harmful organisms.

**Emollient.** A substance that moistens and protects the skin and soothes inflammation, generally in the form of a creamy lotion made from water, oils and wax.

**Emulsifier.** A substance that will produce an emulsion from a combination of liquids.

**Emulsion.** A mixture of liquids that are not soluble in each other but form a suspension, that is one liquid in the form of minute globules suspended in the other.

**Essential oils.** Concentrated essences extracted from aromatic plants which contain the perfumes and other properties of the plant. They have strong therapeutic properties and are used in cosmetics, perfumes and flavourings.

**Exfoliation.** The separation and removal of surface skin by peeling or flaking.

**Hair follicle.** A small cavity in the skin from which the hair grows.

**Glycerine or Glycerol.** A syrupy, colourless, odourless liquid with a sweet taste, extracted from natural fats and oils. It is used in a wide variety of products including as a preservative or sweetener in food and as a skin emollient in the cosmetics industry.

**Infusion.** Herbs steeped in water to obtain an extract used medicinally and cosmetically, internally or externally. Unlike a decoction, the herbs are not boiled in water, therefore this method is adopted for leaves and flowers with more volatile properties.

**Kaolin.** A very fine powder made from the purest form of clay. It is mainly used in face packs to counter oily skin.

**Lecithin.** A coarse fatty powder, extracted from soybeans, egg yolks or corn. It is used in lotions as an emulsifier and also for its important nourishing properties.

**Maceration.** A method of extracting active ingredients from aromatic plants. The plants are steeped in oil, vinegar or pure alcohol. The mixture is left in bottles for two weeks, shaken daily. The strained liquid will keep well. A good method for those plants whose properties are so volatile they would be lost through heating.

**Moisturizer.** A substance that adds or restores water or moisture to the skin.

**Poultice.** A soft, damp compress applied hot to an inflamed or sore part of the body.

**Proteolysis/Proteolytic.** The breaking down of protein into simpler compounds, as occurs during digestion.

**Reactive seborrhea.** An abnormal rate of discharge of oil from the sebaceous glands, as a result of overstimulation from excessive washing.

**Sebaceous duct.** A gland that excretes oily matter to lubricate the skin and hair.

# Index of botanical names

*The English and botanical or Latin names of the plants used in this book.*

| | |
|---|---|
| Agar-agar | *Gelidium* |
| Alkanet | *Alkanna tinctoria* (L.) Tausch |
| Almond | *Prunus dulcis* (Miller) D.A. Webb |
| Aloe | *Aloë* sp. pl. |
| Anise | *Pimpinella anisum* L. |
| Annatto | *Bixa orellanna* L. |
| Apple | *Malus domestica* Borkh |
| Apricot | *Prunus armeniaca* L. |
| Artichoke | *Cynara scolymus* L. |
| Avocado | *Persea gratissima* Gaertn |
| | |
| Balm (lemon) | *Melissa officinalis* L. |
| Banana | *Musa paradisiaca* L. |
| Basil | *Ocimum basilicum* L. |
| Bay (sweet) | *Laurus nobilis* L. |
| Beetroot | *Beta vulgaris* L. |
| Benzoin | *Styrax benzoin* Dryan |
| Birch (silver) | *Betula alba* L. |
| Black currant | *Ribes nigrum* L. |
| Black poplar | *Populus nigra* L. |
| Bladderwrack | *Fucus vesiculosus* L. |
| Butcher's broom | *Ruscus aculeatus* L. |
| | |
| Cabbage | *Brassica oleracea* L. |
| Chamomile (German) | *Camomilla recutita* L. Rauschert |
| Chamomile (Roman) | *Chaemomelum nobile* (L.) All. |
| Camphor | *Cinnamonum canphora* Nees et Eberm |
| Carrot | *Daucus carota* L. |
| Catechu | *Acacia catechu* Wild |
| Cedar of Lebanon | *Cedrus libani* A. Richard |
| Cherry | *Prunus cerasus* L. |
| Chervil | *Anthriscus cerefolium* (L.) Hoffm. |
| Chestnut (horse-) | *Aesculus hippocastanum* L. |
| Chestnut (sweet) | *Castanea sativa* Miller |
| Cinchona | *Cinchona* sp. pl. |
| Clove | *Eugenia caryophyllata* Tunberg |
| Club moss | *Lycopodium clavatum* L. |
| Coffee | *Coffea arabica* L. |
| Coriander | *Coriandrum sativum* L. |
| Cornflower | *Centaurea cyanus* L. |
| Cucumber | *Cucumis sativus* L. |
| Cypress (Mediterranean) | *Cupressus sempervirens* L. |
| | |
| Dandelion | *Taraxacum officinale* Weber |
| Dead-nettle (white) | *Lamium album* L. |
| | |
| Elder | *Sambucus nigra* L. |
| Elm | *Ulmus campestris* L. |
| Eucalyptus | *Eucalyptus globulus* Labill. |
| Evening primrose | *Oenothera biennis* L. |

| | |
|---|---|
| Fennel | *Foeniculum officinale* Allioni |
| Fenugreek | *Trigonella foenum-graecum* L. |
| Fig | *Ficus carica* L. |
| Fir (silver) | *Abies alba* Miller |
| Flax | *Linum usitatissimum* L. |
| | |
| Gentian (yellow) | *Gentiana lutea* L. |
| Ginseng | *Aralla ginseng* Baill. |
| | |
| Helichrysum | *Helichrysum italicum* G. Don. |
| Henna (Egyptian) | *Lawsonia inermis* L. |
| Honeysuckle | *Lonicera caprifolium* L. |
| Hop | *Humulus lupulus* L. |
| Horse-chestnut | *Aesculus hippocastanum* L. |
| Horsetail | *Equisetum arvense* L. |
| | |
| Iceland moss | *Cetraria islandica* (L.) Ach. |
| Indigo | *Indigofera tinctoria* L. |
| Iris | *Iris florentina* L. |
| Ivy | *Hedera helix* L. |
| | |
| Java jute | *Hibiscus sabdariffa* L. |
| Jojoba | *Simmondsia californica* Nutt. |
| Juniper | *Juniperus communis* L. |
| | |
| Kidney vetch | *Anthyllis vulneraria* L. |
| | |
| Laurel: see Bay | |
| Lavender | *Lavandula angustifolia* Miller |
| Lemon | *Citrus limon* (L.) Burm. F. |
| Lemon balm | *Melissa officinalis* L. |
| Lemon verbena | *Lippia citriodora* L. |
| Lettuce | *Lactuca serriola* L. |
| Licorice | *Glycyrrhiza glabra* L. |
| Lily (Madonna) | *Lilium candidum* L. |
| Lime/Linden | *Tillia europaea* L. var. *platyphylla* Scopoli |
| Logwood | *Haematoxylon campechianum* L. |
| Lupin (white) | *Lupinus albus* L. |
| | |
| Madder | *Rubia tinctorium* L. |
| Mallow (common) | *Malva sylvestris* L. |
| Marigold | *Calendula officinalis* L. |
| Marjoram | *Origanum majorana* L. |
| Marsh mallow | *Althea officinalis* L. |
| Meadowsweet | *Filipendula ulmaria* (L.) Maxim. |
| Mediterranean cypress | *Cupressus sempervirens* L. |
| Melilot | *Melilotus officinalis* L. |
| Melon (musk) | *Cucumis melo* L. |
| Melon (water) | *Cucumis citrullus* Ser. |
| Myrrh | *Commiphora molmol* Endl. |
| Myrtle | *Myrtus communis* L. |
| | |
| Nettle (stinging) | *Urtica dioica* L. |
| | |
| Oak (common/English) | *Quercus robur* L. |
| Orange (Seville/bitter) | *Citrus aurantium* L. |
| Orange (common/sweet) | *Citrus sinensis* (L.) Osbeck |
| Oregano | *Origanum vulgare* L. |
| | |
| Papaya | *Carica papaya* L. |
| Parsley | *Petroselinum hortense* Hoffm. |

INDEX OF BOTANICAL NAMES

| | |
|---|---|
| Peach | *Prunus persica* (L.) |
| Pear | *Pyrus communis* L. |
| Pepper | *Piper nigrum* L. |
| Peppermint | *Mentha piperita* L. |
| Pine (Swiss mountain) | *Pinus montana* Miller |
| Pineapple | *Bromelia ananas* L. |
| Plum | *Prunus domestica* L. |
| Plantain | *Plantago major* L. |
| Pomegranate | *Punica granatum* L. |
| Poplar (black, Lombardy) | *Populus nigra* L. |
| Poppy (field) | *Papaver rhoeas* L. |
| Potato | *Solanum tuberosum* L. |
| Primrose (see Evening) | |
| Pumpkin: see also Winter squash | *Cucurbita maxima* Duchesne |
| Psyllium (fleawort) | *Plantago psillium* L. |
| | |
| Quebracho | *Quercus petraea* (Mattuschka) Liebl. |
| | |
| Red currant | *Ribes rubrum* L. |
| Rhubarb | *Rheum officinale* H. Br. |
| Rose | *Rosa* sp. pl. |
| Rose (apothecary's/red) | *Rosa gallica* L. |
| Rosemary | *Rosmarinus officinalis* L. |
| | |
| Safflower | *Carthamus tinctorius* L. |
| Saffron | *Crocus sativus* L. |
| Sage | *Salvia officinalis* |
| St. John's wort | *Hypericum perforatum* L. |
| Sandalwood (red) | *Pterocarpus santalinus* L. |
| Sandalwood (white) | *Santalum album* L. |
| Senna (neutral henna) | *Cassia obovata* |
| Shea (tree) | *Butyrospermum parkii* Kotzkji |
| Silver birch | *Betula alba* L. |
| Silver fir | *Abies alba* Miller |
| Soapbark | *Quillaja saponaria* Molina |
| Soapwort | *Saponaria officinalis* L. |
| Spinach | *Spinacia oleracea* L. |
| Stinging nettle | *Urtica dioica* L. |
| Strawberry | *Fragaria vesca* L. |
| Sweet chestnut | *Castanea sativa* Miller |
| | |
| Tansy | *Tanacetum vulgare* L. |
| Tea | *Thea sinensis* L. |
| Thyme | *Thymus vulgaris* L. |
| Tomato | *Lycopersicum esculentum* Miller |
| Tormentil | *Potentilla erecta* (L.) Rauschel |
| Turmeric | *Curcuma longa* L. |
| | |
| Vine | *Vitis vinifera* |
| | |
| Walnut | *Juglans regla* L. |
| Watercress | *Nasturtium officinale* R. Br. |
| Watermelon | *Cucumis citrullus* Ser. |
| White dead-nettle | *Lamium album* L. |
| Wild strawberry | *Fragaria vesca* L. |
| Winter squash | *Cucurbita maxima* Duchense |
| Witch hazel | *Hamamelis virginiana* L. |
| Woodruff (sweet) | *Galium odoratum* (L.) Scop. |
| | |
| Yarrow | *Achillea millefolium* L. |
| Yellow gentian | *Gentiana lutea* L. |

INDEX OF BOTANICAL NAMES

# Bibliography

Bremness, Lesley *The Complete Book of Herbs* Dorling Kindersley, London 1988

Bryan, John E. & Coralie Castle *The Edible Ornamental Garden* 101 Productions, San Francisco 1974

Buchman, Dian Dincin *Feed Your Face* Duckworth & Co. Ltd., London 1973

Clark, Linda *Secrets of Health and Beauty* Pyramid Books, New York 1970

Genders, Roy *Natural Beauty* Webb & Bower, London 1986

Grieve, Mrs M. *A Modern Herbal* Peregrine, London 1976

Hall, Dorothy *The Book of Herbs* Angus & Robertson, London 1972

Heffern, Richard *The Herb Buyer's Guide* Pyramid Books, New York 1973

Hilker, Li *Beautiful By Nature* David & Charles, London 1989

Horrocks, Lorna *Natural Beauty* Angus & Robertson Publishers, London 1980

Little, Kitty *Kitty Little's Book of Herbal Beauty* Penguin, London 1981

Lust, John *The Herb Book* Bantan, New York 1974

Mabey, Richard *Plants with a Purpose* Collins, London 1977

Maxwell-Hudson, Clare *The Natural Beauty Book* Macdonald, London 1983

Palmer, Catherine *Beauty For Free* Jonathan Cape, London 1981

Rose, Jeanne *Kitchen Cosmetics* North Atlantic Books, Berkeley 1978

# Index

## SUPPLIERS

The following is a list of suppliers who carry many of the ingredients and materials referred to in this book.

**U.S.**
(All take mail order and accept out-of-state orders.)

**Aphrodisia**
282 Bleeker Street
New York, NY 100014
(212) 989-6440

**Arsenic and Old Lace**
1743 Mass Avenue
Cambridge, MA 02140
(617) 354-7785

**Bee Creek Botanicals**
P.O. Box 12006
Austin, TX 78711
(512) 331-4244

**Enchantments, Inc.**
341 East 9th Street
New York, NY 10003
(212) 228-4394

**Fredericksburg Farm**
P.O. Door 927
Fredericksburg, TX 78624-0927
(512) 997-8615

**Greenfield Herb Garden**
P.O. Box 437
Shipshewana, IN 46565
(219) 768-7110

**Greentree Grocers**
3560 Mt. Acadia Blvd.
San Diego, CA 92111
(619) 560-1975

**Herbal Effect**
616 Lighthouse Avenue
Monterey, CA 93940
(408) 375-6313

**Herb Products Co.**
11012 Magnolia Blvd.
North Hollywood, CA 91601
(213) 877-3104

**The HerbFarm**
32804 Issaquah-Fall City Road
Fall City, WA 98024
(206) 784-2222

**Herbs, Etc.**
323 Aztec Street
Santa Fé, NM 87501
(505) 982-1265

**Rathdowney, Ltd.**
P.O. Box 357
Bethel, VT 05032
(802) 234-9928

**San Francisco Herb & Natural Food/Nature's Herb Company**
1010 46th Street
Emeryville, CA 94608
(415) 547-6345

**The Soap Opera**
319 State Street
Madison, WI 53703

**Woodspirits Herb Shop**
1920 Apple Road
St. Paris, OH 43072
(513) 663-4327

**U.K.**

**Baldwins**
173 Walworth Road, London SE17

**Body Treats**
15 Approach Road, Raynes Park, London SW20 8BA

**Culpeper Limited**
Hadstock Road, Linton, Cambridgeshire CB1 6NJ

**Findhorn Apothecary**
The Park, Forres, Scotland IU36 0TY

**Herbs in Stock**
Whites Hill, Stock, Essex CM4 9QB

**Peter Jarvis**
9 Duke Street, Hadleigh, Ipswich, Suffolk

**Neal's Yard Apothecary**
2 Neal's Yard, London WC2

**Potters (Herbal Supplies Limited)**
Leyland Mill Lane, Wigan, Lancs.

**Suffolk Herbs Limited**
Sawyer's Farm, Little Cornard, Sudbury, Suffolk CO10 0NY

The Publisher wishes to thank the following for their collaboration: Brieart (antique furniture and glass), Milan; Moscova Libri e Robe (silver dressing-table set and antique lace), Milan; Musa Ceramiche (decorated and terracotta tiles), Milan; Profumo (bathroom accessories), Milan.